The Top 50

Lifesaving Secrets of the World's Greatest Doctors

Bottom Line Publications

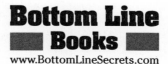

www.BottomLineSecrets.com

BUH/js

Contents

The Top 50 Lifesaving Secrets of the World's Greatest Doctors

Nobel Prize Winner's Breakthrough—Prevent Heart Attack and Stroke With Nitric Oxide

One small molecule produced by the body may do more than any drug to prevent heart attack and stroke. Nitric oxide, a gas that occurs naturally in the body, is critical for healthy circulation. It helps dilate blood vessels, prevent blood clots and regulate blood pressure, and it may inhibit the accumulation of arterial plaque.

HOW IT WORKS

Nitric oxide is a signaling molecule primarily produced by cells in the endothelium (inner lining) of blood vessels. A signaling molecule fits into docking sites (receptors) on cell walls and triggers biochemical reactions. *Nitric oxide helps prevent heart disease and stroke by...*

• **Expanding blood vessels.** Nitric oxide protects the blood vessels' smooth muscle tissue from harmful constriction, and this allows blood to circulate with less force. Some doctors report that elevating nitric oxide in hypertensive patients can lower blood pressure by 10 to 60 points.

• **Controlling platelet function.** Platelets, cell-like structures in blood that can clump up together, may form blood-blocking clots, the main cause of heart attack and stroke. A vascular network that is enhanced by nitric oxide sheds platelets and inhibits dangerous clots.

• **Reducing arterial plaque by 50%.** Arterial plaque, which consists of fatty deposits in the coronary arteries, is the underlying cause of heart disease. Nitric oxide is an antioxidant that inhibits the passage of monocytes, a type of immune cell, into the artery wall. This in turn reduces the underlying inflammation that promotes plaque.

• **Lowering total cholesterol by 10% to 20%.** That's a modest decrease—but there is

Louis J. Ignarro, PhD, winner of the 1998 Nobel Prize in Physiology or Medicine for his research on nitric oxide. He is also a distinguished professor of pharmacology at the University of California, Los Angeles, David Geffen School of Medicine, and author of *No More Heart Disease.* St. Martin's.

some evidence that nitric oxide is even more effective when combined with the cholesterol-lowering statins. Nitric oxide lowers cholesterol through its antioxidant activity. The preliminary research suggests that stimulating nitric oxide production in people who have elevated cholesterol makes it possible to lower their statin doses by at least 50%.

TO BOOST NITRIC OXIDE LEVELS

It is not yet known how much nitric oxide normally is present in the body or what levels are optimal. This gas is difficult to measure because it disappears almost instantly upon exposure to air. Research scientists can measure levels with electrodes inserted in blood vessels. Simpler tests are needed before doctors can measure nitric oxide as part of standard checkups.

Beginning in early adulthood, nitric oxide levels gradually decline, probably due to damage to the endothelial cells caused by such factors as a high-fat diet and a sedentary lifestyle.

Nitric oxide can't be taken in supplement form because it is a gas. However, patients can take other supplements that increase production of nitric oxide in the blood vessels. *These supplements, all available at health-food stores, have few if any side effects…*

• **L-arginine,** an amino acid found in meats, grains and fish, passes through the intestine into the blood. From the blood, it enters endothelial cells, where it is used to make nitric oxide.

A Mayo Clinic study found that people taking L-arginine showed significant improvement in endothelial function and blood flow compared with those taking placebos. It is hard to get sufficient L-arginine from food, so supplements are recommended.

Dose: 2,000 to 3,000 milligrams (mg) taken twice daily—for a total of 4,000 to 6,000 mg.

• **L-citrulline.** Supplemental arginine doesn't enter cells readily unless it is combined with L-citrulline, another amino acid. Melons and cucumbers are rich sources of L-citrulline, but they don't provide high enough levels to significantly increase nitric oxide levels.

Dose: 400 to 600 mg daily.

• **Daily multivitamin that includes vitamin E.** Vitamin E helps reduce the assault of cell-damaging free radicals on the endothelial lining and may promote higher levels of nitric oxide. The amount of vitamin E that is in most multivitamin/mineral supplements is about 50 international units (IU), an effective dose.

Warning: Don't take the high-dose vitamin E supplements. Recent studies suggest that people who take daily doses of 400 IU or higher may be more susceptible to heart disease and other illnesses.

• **Vitamin C.** Like vitamin E, vitamin C will reduce oxidation in the blood vessels and may cause an increase in nitric oxide. People who consume high levels of vitamin C experience a reduction in arterial plaque, which is associated with higher levels of nitric oxide. You can get your vitamin C from food, but I recommend supplements because they are so convenient and easy to take.

Dose: 500 mg daily.

DIET AND EXERCISE

In addition to taking supplements, it is important to maintain a healthy lifestyle by watching what you eat and being active. *Try to…*

• **Do aerobic exercise for at least 20 minutes three days a week.** This stimulates endothelial cells to continuously produce nitric oxide, even on days that you don't exercise.

• **Minimize intake of saturated fat.** Saturated fat, found in such animal products as red meat, poultry, butter and whole milk, contributes to the accumulation of arterial plaque and impairs nitric oxide production.

Better: Olive oil, fish and flaxseed. The fats found in these foods help protect the endothelium by elevating levels of beneficial HDL cholesterol and lowering the harmful LDL form.

• **Eat more fiber.** The dietary fiber in grains, fruits and vegetables lowers blood pressure and LDL cholesterol and raises HDL, thereby protecting endothelial cells.

Bonus: Many of the foods that contain fiber also are rich in antioxidants, which inhibit the cell damage that lowers nitric oxide. Eat at least 25 grams (g) of fiber daily—and drink at least eight 8-ounce glasses of water each day to make sure that the fiber moves through your system properly.

How to Prevent a Heart Attack

People who ate two to three kiwifruits daily for 28 days decreased their platelet aggregation response (potential for blood clot formation) by 18% and their blood triglyceride (fat) levels by 15% compared with people who ate no kiwi. The fruit is rich in polyphenols (antioxidant plant chemicals), vitamins C and E, magnesium, potassium and copper, all of which protect the blood vessels and heart. Kiwifruits are available in grocery stores year-round and can be peeled, sliced and added to green or fruit salads.

Asim K. Duttaroy, PhD, professor of nutritional medicine, department of nutrition, University of Oslo, Norway.

Five Little-Known Ways to Lower Heart Attack Risk

Michael Mogadam, MD, clinical associate professor of medicine at George Washington University School of Medicine in Washington, DC. He is author of *Every Heart Attack Is Preventable: How to Take Control of the 20 Risk Factors and Save Your Life*. New American Library.

Most Americans know all of the traditional heart disease risk factors—lack of physical activity, high cholesterol, high blood pressure, diabetes, obesity and smoking. Although these are important, there also are lesser-known risk factors. *Ways to avoid them...*

•**Boost your HDL level.** Though high LDL ("bad") cholesterol has long been considered the major culprit in heart attack risk, low HDL ("good") cholesterol actually is the bigger risk factor, especially in women. About 70% of women and half of all men with coronary artery disease (CAD) have low HDL cholesterol.

What to do: If you're a woman with HDL below 55 or a man with HDL below 45, take steps to boost your good cholesterol. Engaging in regular, vigorous exercise can raise HDL levels by 10% to 15%. Limiting carbohydrates to less than 45% of your daily diet and increasing monounsaturated fats (which are found in olive, canola and hazelnut oils) can raise HDL levels by 10%. Cholesterol-lowering statin drugs also may raise HDL levels by as much as 10%. Taking 1,500 milligrams (mg) of the B vitamin niacin under the supervision of a health-care provider can raise HDL by 25% to 30%.

Note: At high doses, niacin can cause side effects, such as flushing, liver problems and irregular heart rhythm.

Warning: Low-fat diets invariably lower HDL levels, which may actually *increase* heart attack risk. To ensure a healthy cholesterol ratio, don't simply eliminate fats from your diet. Monounsaturated and nonhydrogenated polyunsaturated fats should provide up to 30% of your total daily calories.

Good sources: Olive oil, canola oil, nuts and avocados.

•**Determine your LDL size.** LDL cholesterol particles come in two sizes—large (type A) and small (type B). A predominance of the type B particles increases risk of CAD by 300% to 500%, *even when LDL levels are normal* (less than 100).

Reason: Small LDL particles pass through the inner lining of coronary arteries more easily, possibly triggering a heart attack.

What to do: If you have low HDL cholesterol levels (below 45 for men and below 55 for women), particularly if any family members developed CAD before age 55, have your LDL particle size measured. This simple blood test is widely available, and many insurers now cover the cost.

The best way to decrease your type-B LDL count is to eat a healthful diet comprised of 30% fat, mostly in the form of monounsaturated fats, and limit carbohydrate intake to no more than 45% of total calories.

To boost your intake of beneficial omega-3 polyunsaturated fats, eat two to three seafood meals weekly. Choose the fattier fish, such as salmon and tuna.

Self-defense: Pregnant and lactating women should ask their doctors about limiting intake of fish due to its mercury content.

Avoid the trans-fatty acids and the omega-6 polyunsaturated fats found in margarine, fried foods, baked goods, corn and safflower oils.

• **Know your birth weight.** A low birth weight is a significant and independent risk factor for heart attack, hypertension and diabetes in adulthood. Research has shown that people who weighed less than 5.5 pounds at birth are three times more likely to develop CAD than people who weighed more than 7.5 pounds at birth.

What to do: Tell your doctor if you had a low birth weight (less than 5.5 pounds)—and show him/her this article. Many health-care providers are unaware of the increased risks associated with low birth weight.

If you were a very small baby, ask your doctor to test regularly for other coronary risk factors, such as hypertension, elevated cholesterol, diabetes and LDL particle size. These factors should be treated aggressively to offset the unalterable risk of low birth weight.

• **Choose heart-healthy beverages.** The heart-protective benefits of alcohol have been well-established. When consumed in moderation (one glass daily for women and no more than two glasses daily for men), wine, beer and mixed drinks reduce CAD by 30%.

Researchers now are discovering that water also may play a role in preventing heart attack. Physicians at Loma Linda University recently reported that drinking five or more glasses of water daily (versus two or fewer) reduces fatal heart attack risk in men by 51% and in women by 35%.

Water seems to protect against heart attacks by making blood less likely to clot. Minerals in hard tap water, such as calcium and magnesium, also may help guard against heart disease.

What to do: Drink from six to eight 8-ounce glasses of water daily. Ask your local water utility if your water is hard (mineral rich) or soft. Even soft water from the tap may be a healthier choice than filtered bottled waters, which are generally stripped entirely of minerals.

Helpful: Consider installing a faucet-mounted home water filter that removes waterborne parasites from your water but doesn't filter out the beneficial minerals.

Good brands: Moen and Culligan.

• **Take folic acid.** This B vitamin has been shown to lower levels of homocysteine, a protein in the blood that significantly increases risk for cardiovascular disease when it is elevated.

Folic acid also lowers the risk for heart attack and stroke.

In continuing research of more than 80,000 nurses, the risk for heart attack was reduced by about 6% for every additional 100 micrograms of folic acid in their diet.

What to do: Eat more folic acid–rich foods, such as spinach, asparagus, lima beans, wheat germ and fortified cereals. If your homocysteine level is greater than 9, you may need to take a folic acid supplement daily.

How to Predict Heart Disease

In a study of more than 72,000 women without infection, those who had the highest levels of white blood cells (WBCs)—6,700 to 15,000—were twice as likely to die from heart disease as women with the lowest levels. Researchers believe this link also applies to men.

Theory: WBC levels, which typically rise in response to infection, also can be a marker for inflammation, which weakens blood vessels and may trigger blockages leading to heart attack or stroke.

Self-defense: Request a WBC count with your next blood test. A level above 6,700 may indicate increased heart disease risk.

Karen L. Margolis, MD, associate professor of medicine, University of Minnesota, Minneapolis.

Cheap, Safe and More Effective Than Statins

Jay S. Cohen, MD, a nationally recognized expert on medications and side effects, his work has been featured in major magazines and on TV programs. He is author of *What You Must Know About Statin Drugs and Their Natural Alternatives* (Square One) and *Over Dose: The Case Against the Drug Companies* (Tarcher-Putnam). His Web site is *www.medicationsense.com*.

First it was on the market, then it was off the market, now it's back on the market. In recent years, the cholesterol-lowering natural supplement *red yeast rice* has sparked many battles among the pharmaceutical companies, the US Food and Drug Administration (FDA) and supplement manufacturers. But in the face of the ongoing controversy regarding statin drugs and how low cholesterol should be, it is good to know about all your options. Red yeast rice is one worth considering.

ABOUT THE CONTROVERSY

In 1998, the FDA yanked red yeast rice, or *monascus purpureus*, from supplement shelves because it contains a natural form of *lovastatin,* the same active ingredient in the patented drug Mevacor. The issue was supposedly one of safety, with prescription statin manufacturers claiming that red yeast rice was an unapproved drug rather than a dietary supplement.

The truth, according to Jay S. Cohen, MD, author of *What You Must Know About Statin Drugs and Their Natural Alternatives*, is that red yeast rice can naturally lower cholesterol levels in the body with fewer side effects and at a considerably lower cost than prescription statins.

However, the FDA didn't see it that way and got onboard with the drug companies. Was red yeast rice taken off the market because of the health risk or because of pharmaceutical company pressures? Or both? Only the FDA knows for sure.

Although the FDA removed it from the market ostensibly to protect the public, critics charge that it actually was the pharmaceutical industry that was being protected from competition from a safer and less-expensive product.

In 1999, a federal judge lifted the ban on red yeast rice products, and today they are available at quality health-food stores.

ASIA'S NATURAL CHOLESTEROL BUSTER

Red yeast rice is made simply by fermenting red yeast on rice. It is commonly consumed as part of the traditional cuisine in China as well as other Asian countries, where people have long believed that it strengthens the heart and circulatory system. Used as a natural food flavoring and coloring agent, it is the ingredient that gives Peking duck its deep red color.

A study at UCLA School of Medicine confirmed red yeast rice's natural cholesterol-busting abilities. In a rigorous double-blind, randomized trial, this supplement significantly reduced total cholesterol compared with a placebo. Among 83 people who took red yeast rice for 12 weeks, total cholesterol dropped by an average of 16% (from approximately 250 to 210)…cholesterol remained at about 250 in the 41 people who were given a placebo. There also was a positive impact on LDL cholesterol and triglyceride levels.

A SAFER ALTERNATIVE

Red yeast rice is a good alternative for people who require mild to moderate cholesterol control but don't want to take statin drugs, says Dr. Cohen. It contains a wide array of cholesterol-lowering compounds, including lovastatin, but all in tiny amounts. This can make it safer than statin drugs and their array of potentially serious side effects, such as liver problems, muscle damage, joint pain, abdominal discomfort and even cognitive or memory problems. According to Dr. Cohen, these effects generally are underestimated and downplayed by the pharmaceutical companies.

EXERCISE CAUTION

Although the amount of lovastatin in red yeast rice is small, it still requires monitoring. Don't take red yeast rice without telling your doctor, and while you are taking it, get checked regularly for liver or muscle problems. Red yeast rice is available in different dosages. The usual recommendation is 1,200 milligrams (mg) daily, divided into two doses. Do not take more than 2,400 mg daily. To reduce the risk for digestive disturbance, take with food.

Some recommendations from the informative manual, *The Physicians' Desk Reference (www. pdrhealth.com)*…

● **Do not take red yeast rice if you have liver disease** or are at risk of developing it, or if you drink more than two alcoholic beverages a day.

● **Do not take this supplement if you are pregnant** or breast-feeding.

● **Do not take red yeast rice if you have a serious infection** or after major surgery.

● **If you develop any muscle pain,** tenderness or twitching, stop using it and consult your doctor.

● **Do not combine red yeast rice with prescription cholesterol-lowering drugs.**

The bottom line? Statins have powerful side effects. Red yeast rice may be a safer alternative for people with mild to moderately high cholesterol. Should you want to try it, it is best to do it under the watchful eye of a physician trained in herbal remedies.

There are many other natural supplements that are helpful for high cholesterol, including plant sterols, inositol hexaniacinate (no-flush niacin), fiber, policosanol, guggulipid, soy and garlic.

The Supplement That Slashes Cholesterol 54% Better Than Statins

Bottom Line's Prescription Alternatives by Earl L. Mindell, RPh, PhD. Bottom Line Books.

Supplements containing policosanol have been found to work well to balance cholesterol counts. Biochemically speaking, policosanol is made up of a series of what's known as fatty alcohols. If you want to know what these *fatty alcohols* naturally look and feel like, scrape a little bit of the waxy film off the leaves of a tree or the peel of a citrus fruit. Commercially sold policosanol supplements are usually made from either sugarcane or beeswax. Citrus peels, wheat germ and caviar are other rich sources of policosanol.

Policosanol has been shown to decrease LDL cholesterol levels by up to 20%, and it increases HDL by an average of 10%—without all the side effects caused by statins. As a matter of fact, in a study of nearly 28,000 people who used policosanol for two to four years, less than half of 1% of the subjects experienced notable adverse effects from their daily dose.

In one study, published in the journal *Gynecology and Endocrinology,* researchers enlisted 244 menopausal women for whom six weeks on a conventional cholesterol-lowering diet did no good. The women were given either a placebo pill or 5 milligrams (mg) of policosanol every day for 12 weeks. The women given policosanol were then given 10 mg for 12 more weeks. By the end of the study, the policosanol users had some amazing changes in their cholesterol levels: Their LDL fell by 25.2%, their total cholesterol fell by 16.7% and their ratio of total cholesterol to HDL fell by 27.2%!

Another study—this one from the *International Journal of Clinical Pharmacology*—compared the effects of policosanol with those of *pravastatin*, a commonly used statin drug, in elderly patients with high cholesterol and high risk of heart attack. These patients took 10 mg of policosanol or pravastatin for eight weeks. Those who took policosanol lowered their LDL by an average of 19.3%...their total cholesterol by an average of 13.9%...and their ratio of total cholesterol to HDL by 24.4%. Pravastatin reduced LDL by only 15.6% and the total cholesterol to HDL ratio by 15.9%, but didn't raise levels of artery-cleaning HDL. In this study, policosanol also stood out for its ability to inhibit the tendency of blood to clot together and clog blood vessels.

Policosanol causes none of the adverse effects statins can cause. It appears to work by slowing the production of cholesterol in the liver while increasing the liver's ability to reabsorb LDL. The most frequently cited side effect? Weight loss—not exactly an undesirable side effect for most people at risk of developing heart disease. Unlike statins, policosanol causes no decrease in libido, and there's a hint of evidence from an animal study that it may actually increase libido slightly! Policosanol also inhibits the oxidation of LDL cholesterol, the free radical attack that makes LDL so much more dangerous to blood vessel health. In animal research, it decreased the uncontrolled inflammation and cell growth known to lead to artery disease. Policosanol also helps to thin the blood, decreasing the chances of a clot forming to plug up an artery and cause a heart attack or stroke.

Levels of a specific type of proinflammatory biochemical called *thromboxane* can rise too high as a direct result of a poor, refined-food diet, and can cause artery walls to clamp down tight, decreasing blood and oxygen flow to the heart and elsewhere. Some studies have shown a decrease in levels of this type of thromboxane with policosanol.

Breakthrough Therapies For Heart Disease, Cancer —and Varicose Veins

Jeff Geschwind, MD, associate professor of radiology, oncology and surgery at Johns Hopkins University School of Medicine, and director of cardiovascular and interventional radiology at The Johns Hopkins Hospital, both in Baltimore.

Heiko Schöder, MD, associate attending physician at Memorial Sloan-Kettering Cancer Center and associate professor of radiology at Weill Medical College of Cornell University, both in New York City.

Sheldon Sheps, MD, cardiologist and emeritus professor of medicine at the Mayo Clinic College of Medicine, Rochester, MN.

Sophisticated radiologic treatments—such as high-speed computed tomography (or CT) scans—now are being used both as an alternative to traditional surgery and as a new diagnostic tool for a number of common ailments.

Typically administered by interventional radiologists, these treatments are available at most medical centers across the US.*

Three leading experts discuss these new therapies below…

CANCER TREATMENT
Jeff Geschwind, MD

When surgical removal of a malignancy of the liver, kidneys, bone or other organs is not an option, due to the size or location of the tumor, patients may now receive a new therapy called *radiofrequency ablation.*

What's involved: An interventional radiologist uses an ultrasound to locate the tumor. A needle is then placed through the skin directly into the malignancy. A radiofrequency current is emitted through the needle to burn away the tumor without damaging any surrounding tissue. The treatment typically takes one to three hours and can be performed as an outpatient procedure, without general anesthesia.

Typical cost: $13,000 to $20,000.

Important: Radiofrequency ablation is only appropriate for the smaller malignancies—that is, tumors no larger than 3 to 4 centimeters (cm) in

*Interventional radiologists specialize in minimally invasive treatments that use image-guided techniques. To find such a specialist in your area, consult the Society of Interventional Radiology (800-488-7284, *www.sirweb.org*).

diameter. This procedure is not a cure for cancer but can be used to help control it.

VARICOSE VEINS

Approximately 25% of all American women and 10% of American men suffer from varicose veins. These will occur when a vein's emptying mechanisms malfunction, resulting in reflux (the pooling of blood), most often in the legs or pelvis. Besides being unsightly, varicose veins also can lead to chronic pain.

A new image-guided technique called *vein ablation,* done with radiofrequency or laser heat, now makes it easier to eradicate varicose veins without surgery or the injection of chemical solutions.

What's involved: Guided by ultrasound, the radiologist threads a small catheter into the varicose vein. The laser is then fired briefly, which heats and seals the vein. The treatment takes less than an hour, and the patient is up and walking 20 minutes later.

Typical cost: $2,000 to $3,000 per leg.

Another new technique uses image-guided therapy to eliminate varicose veins in the pelvis. Some nine million American women suffer from unexplained chronic pelvic pain.

Pelvic congestion syndrome is a condition that has traditionally been very difficult to diagnose and thought to be untreatable. Doctors now believe that many of these cases are triggered by varicose veins in the pelvis.

A *venogram* allows doctors to identify varicose veins in the pelvis. During this procedure, a catheter is inserted and threaded through the affected vein, and an X-ray dye is injected to highlight the vein. An X ray is then taken. Next, small steel coils are implanted to block blood flow through the abnormal vein. This causes the varicose veins to shrivel and disappear.

Typical cost: $7,000.

MALIGNANCY DETECTION
Heiko Schöder, MD

A new technology, known as PET-CT fusion, allows doctors to pinpoint the precise location of cancer cells in the body (for all types of cancer) without having to rely on additional imaging procedures and examinations. The positron emission tomography (PET) locates the small lesions, and the CT scan then precisely pinpoints them.

What's involved: The patient first undergoes a CT scan, a computer-enhanced X-ray study that produces two-dimensional images. Then the patient undergoes a PET scan. For this test, a radioactive substance that's called a "tracer" is injected into a vein. The patient next is placed inside a ring-shaped PET scanner, which detects radiation and records sites of high activity, where cancer is likely to be present. The two tests take about one-half hour to perform. Afterward, the radiologist "fuses" the results of a PET scan with the detailed anatomical images of a CT scan.

Typical cost: $2,000 to $4,000 for both.

A study at Memorial Sloan-Kettering Cancer Center found that the use of combined scans improved accuracy by 42% when diagnosing the location of tumors osf the head and neck.

CORONARY ARTERY DISEASE
Sheldon Sheps, MD

A new five-minute, noninvasive imaging test known as an *electron beam* CT (or EBCT) heart scan can assess the amount of calcium in your coronary arteries. Because calcium is a primary component of arterial plaque, a high coronary calcium level indicates significant plaque build-up in the blood vessels.

What's involved: A cardiologist or radiologist uses the recently developed ultrafast-CT scanner that provides detailed pictures of your heart. The procedure exposes the patient to relatively low levels of radiation.

Typical cost: $400.

A heart scan provides a quick and accurate assessment of heart attack risk without the potential risks associated with an angiogram, in which a catheter is used to inject a dye into the heart that can be seen on X rays.

Surprising Stroke Risks Even Doctors Overlook

Gregory W. Albers, MD, professor of neurology and neurological sciences at Stanford University Medical Center and director of the Stanford Stroke Center.

Stroke is the second most common cause of brain damage (after Alzheimer's disease) and the third most common cause of death (after heart attack and cancer).

Most of us know that risk of stroke can be reduced by controlling high blood pressure and cholesterol, eating a well-balanced diet and exercising on a regular basis. But it is what you may *not* know about this disabling disorder that could save your life.

Often overlooked stroke risks…

PREHYPERTENSION

Until just recently, blood pressure less than 140/90 was considered normal. However, studies now indicate that a reading of 120/80 or higher raises the risk for stroke and should be treated with a combination of exercise, diet and medication, if needed.

What you may not know: Although diuretics, beta blockers and ACE inhibitors have long been utilized to lower blood pressure, recent research reveals that a newer class of antihypertensive medication, called *angiotensin II receptor blockers* (ARBs), may provide unique protection against stroke.

Recent study: An ARB known as *losartan* (Cozaar) reduced stroke risk by an additional 25% over the beta blocker *atenolol* (Tenormin). Several large trials are under way to further study ARBs. If the results are as promising as this preliminary one, ARBs could become the antihypertensive medication of choice for preventing stroke.

Bonus: ARBs cause fewer side effects than other blood pressure medications.

Self-defense: If you take a blood pressure–lowering medication, ask your physician if an ARB would be appropriate for you.

ATRIAL FIBRILLATION

This heart rhythm disturbance affects two million Americans. With atrial fibrillation (AF), the upper chambers of the heart quiver rapidly or irregularly and fail to pump efficiently.

What you may not know: Each year, up to 70,000 strokes are caused by AF. During AF, some patients experience a racing heart, palpitations or a fluttering in their chest, dizziness and/or shortness of breath. For other patients, the first symptom of AF may be a stroke.

Self-defense: To determine if you may have AF, put your index finger on your wrist and check your pulse for an irregular or random rhythm. AF can be confirmed with a routine electrocardiogram (EKG).

If you are diagnosed with AF, your doctor may prescribe an antiarrhythmic medication, such as *digoxin* (Lanoxin) or *amiodarone* (Cordarone), or a type of electric shock, known as cardioversion, to correct the arrhythmia.

However, the recurrence rate for AF is high with these therapies. It is usually preferable to choose a treatment that prevents blood clots, rather than focusing on the heart rhythm disturbance. Lifetime use of anticoagulants can reduce stroke risk in AF patients by 68%.

The most frequently prescribed anticoagulant, *warfarin* (Coumadin), is extremely effective at preventing clots and reducing stroke risk in people with AF. Unfortunately, it has a narrow "therapeutic index"—slightly too much in your system can cause bleeding…slightly too little will permit stroke.

Warfarin also interacts with other drugs, supplements and even foods.

Example: Vitamin K, which is found in the leafy greens and margarine, counteracts the effects of warfarin.

Because warfarin does interfere with so many common substances, people taking it need to undergo monthly blood tests…and physicians must adjust the dosage frequently. As a result, less than half of AF patients who should take Coumadin actually do.

The anticoagulant called *ximelagatran* (Exanta) looked promising as a way to revolutionize stroke and blood clot prevention. However, it was recently withdrawn from the market due to reports of serious liver problems in a clinical trial.

LEG PAIN

Just as atherosclerosis can narrow blood vessels to the heart and brain, it also can block arteries in the extremities, causing peripheral artery disease (PAD). Leg pain—especially in the calves—is the chief symptom. Known as intermittent claudication, the pain typically begins with walking and ends when you stop. PAD affects up to 20% of Americans who are age 65 or older.

What you may not know: If you have PAD, you also may have atherosclerosis elsewhere in the body, such as the heart or the brain. This puts you at increased risk for stroke. What's more, you also can have "silent," or asymptomatic, PAD. Risk factors for PAD are the same as those for cardiovascular disease—high blood pressure, high cholesterol, diabetes, smoking, age, etc.

Self-defense: PAD is easily and painlessly diagnosed with an ankle brachial index test, which measures the ratio of blood pressure in the arm and ankle.

If you're diagnosed with PAD, your physician might prescribe an antiplatelet medication, such as aspirin or *clopidogrel* (Plavix). Moderate exercise to reduce leg pain and blood pressure or cholesterol-lowering medications also may be recommended.

SLEEP APNEA

This disorder occurs when breathing is temporarily interrupted during sleep. An estimated 24% of men and 9% of women suffer from significant sleep apnea.

What you may not know: People with sleep apnea are three to six times more likely to suffer a stroke. Their blood pressure increases dramatically during the night, which can raise the risk for atherosclerotic blockages of the carotid—or neck—arteries, and this is a chief cause of stroke.

In one recent study involving men ages 45 to 77, more than 21% of patients with sleep apnea had calcified plaques, which block blood flow, in their carotid arteries. Only 2.5% of the healthy control patients had calcified plaques.

Self-defense: Obesity is the leading risk factor for sleep apnea…and loud snoring and excessive daytime sleepiness are telltale signs. If you suspect you may have sleep apnea, consult your physician about diagnosis and the best treatment options.

Caution: It's important for AF patients who have symptoms of sleep apnea to undergo sleep apnea screening. Mayo Clinic researchers recently reported that AF is twice as likely to recur in patients with untreated sleep apnea.

Latest Developments In Stroke Rehab

Michael Reding, MD, associate professor of neurology at Weill Medical College of Cornell University, New York City. He is director of stroke rehabilitation at the Burke Rehabilitation Hospital, White Plains, NY.

Most stroke patients require rehabilitation to recover their physical skills and to regain the ability to live independently.

Recent developments in stroke rehabilitation are now helping patients recover better and faster, sometimes even several years after the stroke.

The following therapies are the latest approaches to stroke recovery. Check with the stroke centers located in your area about what is available.

ARMS AND LEGS

Stroke patients often require physical therapy for arm or leg weakness or immobility. Repetitive physical movements prevent muscle atrophy and enhance the brain cells in the area surrounding the stroke damage. *Breakthrough therapies...*

•**Robotic therapy.** MIT researchers have developed the tabletop robot MIT-Manus, which significantly improves arm mobility—and may be even more effective than conventional physical therapy.

How it works: The patient puts his/her lower arm and wrist into a brace attached to the robot. A video screen prompts the patient to perform arm exercises, such as connecting dots on the screen. The robot monitors movement and increases or decreases resistance as required—and even moves the arm if the patient is unable to do so. The robot can move the arm thousands of times in a single session and detects (and responds to) movements and muscle tension that are too subtle for the patient to notice.

Patients who use robotic therapy have muscle strength scores that are about twice as high as those undergoing traditional physical therapy.

Most patients enjoy the interactive nature of this "video game" therapy. It gives immediate feedback and boosts their motivation to keep trying. Between 18 and 36 sessions are needed.

•**Bilateral arm training with rhythmic auditory cueing (BATRAC).** When patients move both the damaged arm and the healthy arm together (bilateral movement), the healthy side of the brain promotes better functioning in the side damaged by stroke.

How it works: The patient works with an occupational therapist for about an hour several days a week. He performs movements to the beat of a metronome or another auditory device. He moves both arms simultaneously—for example, moving arms away from the body, then moving them back in.

Early studies indicate that patients treated with BATRAC have greater improvements in upper-extremity motor function than those who are treated with conventional therapy.

•**Constraint-induced movement therapy.** When a stroke victim has trouble moving a limb, damage to the brain's sensory cortex may cause him to lose awareness of that hand, arm or leg—and he stops moving it entirely.

How it works: In constraint-induced therapy, placing the healthy limb in a sling forces the patient to use the disabled limb, thereby facilitating the regaining of movement control. This approach requires the patient to practice for up to six hours a day for several weeks.

For example, he might be asked to pick up a block of wood, sweep floors, throw balls or draw pictures repeatedly.

The therapy is performed in a clinic setting, often in groups to encourage participation and enhance motivation.

Studies have shown that this approach results in improvements in motor function and muscle strength.

WALKING

Patients who are in conventional rehabilitation programs typically use canes or leg braces for support.

For safety reasons, they walk slowly, and they may not reach their optimal level of recovery.

•**Body weight support.** With body weight support, patients can more than double their speed.

Faster walking hastens recovery and prepares patients for the types of movements they will need in daily life, such as quickly crossing a street.

How it works: The patient is suspended in a harness attached to a weight-support system. The harness prevents the patient from falling, so he can increase the speed of the treadmill and push himself harder. The harness adjusts to support more or less of the patient's body weight, depending on his progress.

SWALLOWING

Many patients experience difficulty swallowing (dysphagia). Traditionally, speech therapists teach patients how to initiate normal swallowing movements.

● **VitalStim treatment.** Electrical stimulation applied to the neck causes the muscles that are involved in swallowing to activate at the appropriate times. This approach is effective in as little as one week.

How it works: Electrodes are placed on the neck. Electrical currents stimulate muscles in the throat to contract. The treatment, lasting 20 to 30 minutes, may be repeated 10 or more times over a week. It retrains the brain to stimulate involuntary swallowing movements.

Drawbacks: This does not work for all patients. Many require speech therapy sessions. Also, the treatment may be uncomfortable—it causes a feeling of tightness in the neck, as though one is being grabbed by the throat.

VISION

● **Visual retraining.** Stroke victims who experience vision damage can receive significant improvement from a technique called visual retraining, or vision restoration therapy.

How it works: The patient fixes his eyes on a spot on a monitor, then clicks a button when he becomes aware that another dot has appeared in the periphery. This stimulates neurons in the visual center of the brain. Sessions usually are 30 minutes, twice daily, for six months.

A study presented at the American Stroke Association International Conference reported that patients were able to detect 62% of the peripheral dots after six months, compared with 54% when they began. Follow-up studies show that 70% of patients maintain the improvement more than a year later.

BEWARE OF DEPRESSION

Depression is common in stroke patients in the first year.

One study found that patients who suffer poststroke depression are 3.5 times more likely to die within 10 years than those who aren't depressed.

Stroke patients should be evaluated for depression and, if diagnosed, given appropriate treatment, which can include psychotherapy and/or antidepressants. Treatment can greatly improve patients' motivation and increase their rate of recovery.

Cancer Vaccines Offer New Hope

Michael Morse, MD, associate professor of medicine in the division of medical oncology at the Duke University Medical Center, Durham, NC. He is editor of *Handbook of Cancer Vaccines*, Humana, and has published more than 150 scientific papers, book chapters and abstracts on immunotherapy. He has also developed several cancer vaccinations.

Until recently, cancer treatment was limited to three options—surgery, chemotherapy and/or radiation.

Now: Cancer *vaccines* are a promising new treatment for virtually all types of malignancies.

To learn more, we spoke with Michael Morse, MD, a medical oncologist and leading authority on cancer vaccines...

● **Is the idea of cancer vaccines new?** Not at all. In the 1700s, it was observed that people with tumors occasionally improved after they experienced an infection. Then, more than a century ago, William Coley, a New York surgeon, identified a patient who had an incurable sarcoma (cancer of the bone, muscle or other supportive tissue) but who experienced a significant reduction of the sarcoma after contracting a skin infection.

Coley then tried treating some patients by injecting them—and their tumors—with a fluid in which two types of bacteria were grown. This was called Coley toxin, which artificially induced inflammation in cancer patients and resulted in an improvement in 40% of patients and a cure in 10%. This treatment, nonspecific *immunotherapy,* activates the immune system in a general way.

In the last 20 years, immunotherapy for cancer, using vaccines to activate the immune system in a specific way, has become an important field of cancer research.

● **How do cancer vaccines work?** Cancer vaccines aren't like vaccines for viral diseases, such as influenza. Although they do not currently *prevent* cancer, we do hope that one day they will. Rather, they use various methods to stimulate the cells of the immune system to attack cancer cells.

A cancer vaccine uses an *antigen,* a protein-based derivative from a tumor. Once inside the body, the antigen is taken up by *dendritic cells,* sentinel-like immune cells that break up the antigen and represent it in a form that T-cells can recognize. These T-cells are stimulated by the dendritic cells to then divide into large numbers and to acquire the capacity to recognize and destroy harmful tumor cells.

Our goal is to trigger the immune system to produce an abundance of these "smart" T-cells that can work to eliminate the malignancy.

•**What kinds of cancer can the vaccines fight?** Virtually every type of cancer has been studied in a clinical trial, including brain cancer. Many of these trials have been conducted with patients who have metastatic, or advanced, disease.

Vaccines are also being used in "adjuvant" settings—in a person who has had a tumor and has a high risk of recurrence. For example, a patient who has been surgically treated for breast cancer may subsequently receive chemotherapy, hormonal therapy *and* a cancer vaccine in a clinical trial to discover if immunotherapy helps make the other two treatments more successful in preventing a recurrence.

Many of these adjuvant studies are focused on melanoma, a deadly skin cancer, because it is thought to be more susceptible to the immune system's attack.

•**How successful are the cancer vaccines?** Studies show that 3% to 5% of solid tumors, such as those found in the lung, breast or prostate, shrink after the use of a cancer vaccine.

In nonsolid, or hematological, cancers, such as leukemias and lymphomas, the response rate is slightly higher, because of the unique antigens in these types of cancers.

These success rates may sound low, but there's reason to be optimistic. Many studies report that a patient whose immune system is successfully activated by the vaccine either lives longer or experiences slower growth of the cancer than someone whose immune system is not successfully activated.

A recent study of the vaccine Theratope, used for breast cancer, did not show a positive result overall but did show benefit in a subgroup of women who were taking hormone therapy, primarily the drug *tamoxifen* (Nolvadex). The median overall survival for patients taking hormonal therapy who received Theratope was 36.5 months, compared with 30.7 months for those who received the control vaccine.

Further clinical trials will focus on the effectiveness of cancer vaccines in these and other subgroups.

Before long, we may learn the best way to give dozens of specifically targeted vaccines to help many kinds of patients.

Researchers also have reason for cautious optimism because these vaccines do work—they generate T-cells that recognize and fight off cancer. Before cancer vaccinations, there were fewer such T-cells.

Even when tumors do not significantly shrink, cancer patients who have an immune response to vaccines have had longer periods before the cancer worsened than non-vaccine patients, and they have survived longer.

•**Are cancer vaccines toxic?** No, not in the same way that chemotherapy can be toxic. Using a vaccine to stimulate the immune system might be thought of as a "natural" way to treat cancer. It does not have the same side effects as those caused by chemotherapy and radiation, but it can cause fevers, allergic reactions and autoimmune disorders.

Cancer patients consider vaccines nontoxic, and that's one reason why they are so excited about the prospect of this treatment.

•**How can people with cancer find out about the availability of cancer vaccines?** Cancer vaccines are being tested but are not yet available as part of the standard treatment regimen offered by cancer specialists.

However, there are more than 150 ongoing clinical trials involving cancer vaccines. Be sure to talk to your oncologist about cancer vaccines to see if this treatment might be available and right for you.

For more information on clinical trials for cancer vaccines, contact the National Cancer Institute at 800-422-6237 or visit its Web site at *www.cancer.gov/clinicaltrials.*

Skin Cancer: Debunking the Myths

Barney J. Kenet, MD, a dermatologist specializing in skin cancer. Dr. Kenet is a dermatologic surgeon at NewYork–Presbyterian Hospital/Weill Cornell Medical Center in New York City, and is coauthor (with Patricia Lawler) of *Saving Your Skin—Prevention, Early Detection, and Treatment of Melanoma and Other Skin Cancers.* Four Walls Eight Windows.

Everyone knows that excessive sun exposure is dangerous, and yet up to 50% of people over age 65 are diagnosed with melanoma or some other type of skin cancer.

Why? Even health-savvy individuals remain confused about the best ways to adequately protect their skin.

Most dangerous myths…

Myth #1: **A beach umbrella keeps you safe from the sun.**

Reality: When you're at the beach, a large percentage of ultraviolet (UV) light bounces off the sand onto your skin, even when you are beneath an umbrella. Water and snow have the same reflective effect.

When boating or sitting beneath the beach umbrella, apply a sunscreen to all the exposed areas, including your face and neck—even if you're wearing a brimmed hat. When skiing, apply sunscreen to your face and neck.

Myth #2: **Sunscreen with a sun-protection factor (SPF) of 45 is three times more effective than SPF 15.**

Reality: Most doctors recommend using a sunscreen with an SPF of at least 15. A higher SPF will not give you much additional protection. A sunscreen that has an SPF of 45 is only about 5% more protective than an SPF 15 sunscreen. The higher-rated sunscreen doesn't last any longer, either.

All sunscreens need to be reapplied every two hours—and whenever you're exposed to water. This includes "waterproof" sunscreens, which provide some protection while swimming but still must be reapplied.

Make sure your sunscreen is labeled "broad spectrum"—meaning that it blocks both ultraviolet A (UVA) and ultraviolet B (UVB) rays. Look for titanium dioxide or Parsol 1789 in the listing of ingredients.

Myth #3: **Sunscreen provides complete sun protection.**

Reality: While sunscreen is essential, there are other steps you also should take. The most important is to minimize sun exposure between 10 am and 4 pm, when the sun's rays are most intense. Hit the beach in the early morning or late afternoon instead.

To protect the commonly neglected areas, be sure to wear…

• UV-protective lip balm with an SPF of 15 or higher.

• A hat with a three-inch brim. Baseball caps don't protect the ears or the back of the neck—common skin cancer sites, especially for golf and tennis players.

• UV-protective sunglasses. Exposure to UV can cause cataracts.

• Sun-protective clothing. UV rays can pass through many fabrics, including cotton. If you hold a garment up to a light and can see the shape of the bulb shining through, it's not providing adequate sun protection.

Many companies offer lightweight, tightly woven garments designed for comfort and maximum protection.

Example: Solumbra 30+ SPF sun protective clothing (800-882-7860, *www.sunprecautions.com*).

If you will be outdoors and don't have special clothing, be sure to wear sunscreen under your shirt.

Myth #4: **Family history is the best indication of skin cancer risk.**

Reality: A family history of skin cancer is a major risk factor—but the most important factor is your own skin type. People who have light-colored skin and eyes (blue or green) and freckles are at highest risk for all types of skin cancer and sun-related skin damage, such as wrinkles.

People with many moles, freckles and spots have the next-highest cancer risk, followed by individuals with a family history of skin cancer. If you have any of these risk factors, you need to carefully monitor your sun exposure.

When the skin is exposed to sunlight, it increases the body's production of *melanin,* the main skin pigment. This results in tanning, in which a brown color is imparted to the skin.

The more difficult it is for you to tan, the more vulnerable you are to skin cancer.

If you're dark-skinned, tan easily, don't have many moles and have no family history of skin cancer, your risk is low but you should still protect yourself from the sun.

Myth #5: **Building a "base" tan protects against sunburn.**

Reality: There is no such thing as a "safe" tan. UV exposure increases lifetime risk of skin cancer and other skin damage. Rather than expose yourself to those pre-vacation rays, protect yourself by following the rules described in this article.

Myth #6: **"Self-tanning" products help protect against sunburn.**

Reality: Self-tanning products are perfectly safe and are a good way to appear tan without any sun exposure.

However, the dyes in these products do not offer UV protection. Some of these products do contain sunblock, but this provides only two hours of protection following application.

Myth #7: **Melanoma occurs only where the skin has been exposed to the sun.**

Reality: Sun exposure is just one of the potential causes of melanoma. For unknown reasons, cancerous moles can also develop under the arm, between the buttocks or toes or on the bottom of the foot.

If you have a mole, spot or freckle *anywhere* on your body that shows a sudden change in size, shape or color, get it checked by a dermatologist.

Myth #8: **Melanoma is always deadly.**

Reality: When limited to the top layers of the skin, melanoma has a cure rate of 100%. That's why it's important to do a monthly self-exam of all skin surfaces, using a full-length and a handheld mirror.

You should also get screened annually by a dermatologist (twice a year, if you have skin cancer risk factors). During the screening, the doctor should use *epiluminescence microscopy* (ELM). This new technique, which involves examining moles with a handheld microscope, detects melanoma earlier than ever.

Prostate Cancer Fighter

In laboratory experiments, disease-fighting flavonoids found in cranberries destroyed human prostate cancer cells.

Theory: Flavonoids interfere with the signals that tell cancer cells to proliferate.

More research is under way to confirm these findings. In the meantime, eat homemade cranberry sauce, snack on whole dried cranberries (sold in supermarkets) and/or drink 100% cranberry juice.

Peter J. Ferguson, PhD, research associate, London Regional Cancer Program, London, Ontario, Canada.

Longevity Boosters From the World's Longest-Lived People

Bradley J. Willcox, MD, investigator in geriatrics and gerontology, Pacific Health Research Institute, and clinical assistant professor of geriatrics, University of Hawaii, both in Honolulu. He is also coauthor of The Okinawa Program: How the World's Longest-Lived People Achieve Everlasting Health—and How You Can Too. Three Rivers Press.

The residents of Okinawa, an island chain of Japan, are among the healthiest and longest-lived people in the world. Okinawa has more 100-year-olds than anywhere else —33.6 per 100,000 people, compared with approximately 10 per 100,000 in the US.

The 25-year Okinawa Centenarian Study discovered that, compared with Americans, Okinawans have...

•**80% lower risk of breast and prostate cancers.**

•**50% lower risk of colon and ovarian cancers.**

•**40% fewer hip fractures.**

•**Minimal risk of heart disease.**

What is the secret to the Okinawans' longevity—and what can we do to achieve the same healthful vigor? *The following factors are especially important...*

ACCEPTING ATTITUDE

While many Americans exhibit Type A personalities, Okinawans believe that life's travails will work themselves out. The average American might be said to suffer from *hurry sickness*. Okinawans prefer to work at their own pace, referred to locally as *Okinawa Time*. They don't ignore stress…but they rarely internalize it.

Stress will signal your body to secrete large amounts of *cortisol* and other stress hormones. That damages the heart and blood vessels and accelerates bone loss.

To reduce stress: Don't take on more than you can handle…take advantage of flextime at work…don't get worked up about things you can't change, such as traffic jams or rude behavior…practice deep breathing and meditation.

LOW-CALORIE INTAKE

Okinawans consume an average of 1,900 calories a day, compared with 2,500 for Americans. Studies have shown that animals given a diet with 40% fewer calories than the diets of free-feeding animals live about 50% longer.

Reason: Harmful oxygen molecules (free radicals) are created every time the body metabolizes food for energy. Because the Okinawans take in fewer calories, their lifetime exposure to free radicals—which damage cells in the arteries, brain and other parts of the body—is reduced.

PLANT-BASED DIET

About 98% of the *traditional* Okinawan diet is made up of sweet potatoes, soy-based foods, grains, fruits and vegetables. All this is supplemented by a small amount of fish (and lean pork on special occasions). These plant foods contain *phytonutrients*—chemical compounds that reduce free radical damage. A plant-based diet is also high in fiber, which lowers cholesterol and reduces the risk of diabetes, breast cancer and heart disease. The *current* Okinawan diet is about 80% plant food.

Wok advantage: The Okinawans' style of cooking is high-heat stir-frying in a wok, which requires little oil. They typically stir-fry with canola oil, which is high in heart-healthy monounsaturated fat and omega-3 fatty acids. These fatty acids lower levels of LDL (bad) cholesterol while increasing levels of HDL (good) cholesterol.

SOY FOODS

Elderly Okinawans eat an average of two servings of soy foods daily—such as tofu, miso soup and soybean sprouts. Soy is rich in flavonoids, chemical compounds that reduce the tendency of LDL to stick to arteries, thereby reducing the risk of heart disease or stroke. Soy foods may also protect against cancer…menopausal discomfort (such as hot flashes)…and osteoporosis. You don't have to eat a lot of soy foods to get similar benefits. One daily serving of tofu (about three ounces) or soy milk (eight ounces) may be protective.

FISH

Fish harvested from the waters surrounding Okinawa is an integral part of the residents' daily diet. The omega-3 fatty acids in fish "thin" the blood and reduce the risk of clots—the main cause of heart attack.

Omega-3s also inhibit the body's production of inflammatory chemicals called *prostaglandins*. That may lower the risk of inflammatory conditions, such as arthritis and the bowel disorder Crohn's disease.

Americans can get similar benefits by eating fish at least three times a week. Cold-water fish —salmon, mackerel, tuna—contain the largest amounts of omega-3s. Fish oil supplements are a worthwhile alternative for people who are "fish phobic."

HEALTHY WEIGHT

The traditional Okinawan diet is low in fat and processed foods, as well as calories—so obesity is rare in elder Okinawans. This means their risk of weight-related health problems, such as diabetes, heart disease and cancer, is much lower than that of Americans. This is in stark contrast to younger Okinawans, who eat a more Westernized diet and have the highest obesity levels in Japan.

Postmenopausal bonus: After menopause, a woman's main source of estrogen is no longer the ovaries, but extraglandular tissues, mainly body fat. Women who maintain a healthful weight produce less estrogen, which reduces the risk for breast cancer.

JASMINE TEA

Okinawans drink about three cups of jasmine tea daily. It contains more antioxidant flavonoids than black tea. Those antioxidants may reduce risk for heart disease as well as some cancers.

NOT SMOKING

In the US, hundreds of thousands of people die from smoking-related diseases annually. Few elderly Okinawans have ever smoked...although one man interviewed for the study took up smoking when he was 100. He got bored with it and quit the next year. About 60% of younger Okinawan men now smoke.

EXERCISE

People are healthiest when they combine aerobic, strengthening and flexibility exercises. Okinawans often get all three by practicing martial arts or a traditional style of dance that resembles tai chi. *Smart regimen...*

• **Swimming,** biking, jogging, etc. for at least 30 minutes three times weekly.

• **Lifting weights** at least 20 minutes twice a week.

• **Flexibility exercises**—yoga or stretching —whenever you can and certainly after each aerobic or strength-training session.

SOCIAL LINKS

Moai is the Okinawan word that means "meeting for a common purpose." Groups of friends, colleagues or relatives get together at least once each month to talk...share gossip...and provide emotional or even financial support.

People who maintain active social networks live longer and are less likely to get sick. When they do get sick, they recover more quickly if they have the support of friends.

SPIRITUALITY AND RELIGION

People who have spiritual or religious beliefs live longer than those who don't. Spirituality and religion are a part of daily life in Okinawa. People pray daily for health and peace. They look out for one another in a "help thy neighbor" ethic called *Yuimaru*. Moderation is a key cultural value.

Women are the religious leaders in Okinawa. They also tend to have very high levels of life satisfaction and respect as they age.

Best Herb for Male Urinary Tract Problems

Whole saw palmetto extract might work even better than standard saw palmetto extract for male urinary tract problems. But, be sure to see a doctor formally trained in botanical medicine before trying any of the herbal medications.

Recommended: The Eclectic Institute's fresh freeze-dried berry extract, Serenoa serrulata (800-332-4372, *www.eclecticherb.com*).

Andrew L. Rubman, ND, director, Southbury Clinic for Traditional Medicines, Southbury, CT, *www.naturopath. org.*

Stop Memory Loss Before It's Too Late

Zaldy S. Tan, MD, MPH, director of the Memory Disorders Clinic at Beth Israel Deaconess Medical Center and instructor in medicine at Harvard Medical School, both in Boston. He is author of *Age-Proof Your Mind: Prevent, Detect, and Stop Memory Loss—Before It's Too Late.* Warner.

Alzheimer's disease, the dread destroyer of memory, doesn't happen all at once. Like heart disease and many other serious ailments, it's years in the making.

Only recently have medical researchers nailed down the early warning signs of Alzheimer's. People who have a condition known as mild cognitive impairment (MCI), which marks the transitional stage between normal aging and dementia, are highly likely to develop Alzheimer's. According to a Mayo Clinic study, 15% of people with MCI have Alzheimer's one year later, compared with 1% to 2% of those without MCI. Within four years, 50% of people with MCI will have Alzheimer's...after five years or longer, it's 80% to 90%.

Can this downward spiral be stopped? As yet, the jury still is out, but there is reason to be hopeful. After all, 10% to 20% of people who have MCI do *not* fall victim to Alzheimer's. What protects them?

A growing body of scientific evidence suggests that staying mentally active, exercising regularly and eating well can help preserve memory—and slow or perhaps even halt the progression of MCI.

NORMAL AGING OR MCI?

People with MCI have the same kind of lapses in short-term memory—forgetting facts, names, appointments, etc.—that most of us experience as we progress through our 50s, 60s and beyond …but many more such instances.

They still remember how to perform everyday activities, such as driving, reading, typing and cooking. Their ability to reason, solve math problems and control emotions also is left intact.

A key criterion for identifying MCI is "subjective" memory loss—that is, the person notices the lapses and thinks that they are troublesome and too frequent. Still, people differ widely in their sensitivity to their own memory performance. Often, friends and family become aware of memory problems before the person experiencing them does. Perhaps the most reliable indicator is performance on memory tests administered by a psychologist, psychiatrist, geriatrician or neurologist.

BRAIN TO SPARE

MCI progresses to Alzheimer's disease when enough brain cells are affected to seriously compromise the brain's ability to function. The more densely interconnected your brain cells are, the greater your "brain reserve." This allows your brain to keep on working well even if some cells have been affected.

Researchers now know that new *synapses*—connections between brain cells—can be formed throughout life.

Mental activity builds synapses the same way physical activity builds muscle. If you are concerned about your memory, it's critical to challenge your mind.

Self-defense: Spend at least one hour daily performing rigorous mental activity. Read books on subjects that demand concentration…do crossword puzzles at a level you find difficult…take an adult education course in a new discipline…work conscientiously to master a foreign language.

YOU CAN HALT MENTAL DECLINE

Mental activity is only part of the story. The same lifestyle and diet changes that are recommended to reduce the risk for heart attack, cancer and other serious diseases maximize brain reserve as well by maintaining brain cells and stimulating the connections between them.

● **Exercise.** Physical activity keeps brain cells well nourished and supplied with the oxygen they need to survive.

A six-year study of 345 Californians age 55 or older found significantly less mental decline among those who were more physically fit than the others.

Self-defense: Any regular exercise you enjoy, even 30 minutes of brisk walking daily, will help.

Ideal: Physical activities that also challenge your mind, such as ballroom dancing or learning a new sport.

● **Limit calories.** One source of free radicals (high-energy oxygen molecules that are known to damage brain cells) is the conversion of food to energy. The more you eat, the more toxic molecules are created.

Human population studies have linked calorie restriction to slower aging. In one study conducted at Columbia University, those who ate the fewest calories had the lowest risk of developing Alzheimer's.

Self-defense: If you're moderately active, aim for 1,800 to 2,200 calories per day.

● **Get your fruits and vegetables.** Foods rich in antioxidant vitamins and similar plant-based chemicals appear to protect brain cells against harmful free radicals.

In a Dutch study, people who consumed more than 23 international units (IU) daily of vitamin E had a 43% reduction in Alzheimer's risk. Similar protection was found in those who consumed 133 mg or more daily of vitamin C.

Self-defense: Include in your daily diet antioxidant-rich foods, such as spinach (one cup provides 10 IU of vitamin E)…or frozen peaches (one cup contains 235 milligrams [mg] of vitamin C).

There is less evidence that antioxidant supplements are protective.

● **Eat fish.** Like the heart, the brain benefits from the omega-3 fatty acids found in fish.

In a Rush University study of more than 800 older adults, the Alzheimer's risk in those who ate fish at least once weekly was 60% lower than in those who did not.

Self-defense: Eat cold-water fish that is high in omega-3 fatty acids—halibut, mackerel or salmon, for example—at least once weekly.

PROTECTIVE MEDICATION?

Research now suggests that inflammation—the same process that causes many diseases, such as rheumatoid arthritis—destroys brain cells. Inflammation-fighting drugs may protect against Alzheimer's disease.

Studies from Mayo Clinic have found a significantly lower incidence of Alzheimer's among people who took nonsteroidal anti-inflammatory drugs (NSAIDs), such as *ibuprofen* (Advil), regularly for at least two years.

Other studies suggest that people who take cholesterol-lowering statin drugs are also less likely to develop the disease.

The evidence is still too weak to justify regular use of NSAIDs or statins for everyone. These drugs have risks—NSAIDs can cause gastrointestinal bleeding and statins can cause side effects, such as muscle pain and liver problems.

If you have MCI, however, the drugs' potential benefits may outweigh the risks. Talk to your doctor.

More from Dr. Zaldy Tan...

Test Your Memory

Ask someone to read aloud a list of four unrelated words, pausing for one second between each.

Examples: Freedom, strawberry, tiger, north ...flower, truck, valor, dentist.

After memorizing the list, perform an unrelated task. Five minutes later, say the words out loud to your companion.

If you missed some, have him/her read them to you again. Five minutes later, repeat the words out loud again and note your score. Do the same 20 minutes after that. Most people will remember all or three of the words.

Because inborn memory ability varies and is influenced by age, education and other factors, there's no "passing grade" on this test. Take the test again four to six months later. If your ability to perform the test declines—particularly if you're

aware of memory problems in the meantime — seek an evaluation.

You Can Prevent Alzheimer's Disease

Majid Fotuhi, MD, PhD, assistant professor of neurology at Johns Hopkins University School of Medicine and director of the Center for Memory and Brain Health at Sinai Hospital, both in Baltimore. He also is clinical instructor in neurology at Harvard Medical School, Boston, and author of *The Memory Cure: How to Protect Your Brain Against Memory Loss and Alzheimer's Disease.* McGraw-Hill.

The scientists who research Alzheimer's disease (or AD) have yet to discover what causes the formation of abnormal protein structures (called plaques and tangles) that destroy brain cells.

However: It's now clear that certain lifestyle practices can guard against the inexorable memory loss and personality changes associated with this dreaded disease.

Evidence: In a landmark study of 678 Midwestern nuns, autopsy reports found that the brains of one-third of the 251 nuns who died in the course of the study had the plaques and tangles of AD but did *not* show symptoms of the disease. On the other hand, some nuns who had *fewer* plaques and tangles had experienced AD symptoms.

ASSAULTS ON THE BRAIN

AD gets the lion's share of attention, but it's just one of many enemies that menace the brain as we grow older. *Among them...*

•**Inflammation.** This is a normal defense mechanism in which the immune system destroys foreign molecules, such as viruses, by releasing high-energy molecules, including free radicals.

With aging, a mild degree of inflammation occurs in joints, skin and the brain, causing arthritis, skin wrinkles and memory problems.

•**Ministrokes.** Each ministroke (blockage of tiny blood vessels within the brain) may kill too few cells to produce any noticeable impact, but when ministrokes occur hundreds—or even thousands—of times, they take their toll.

It is the *cumulative* impact that counts—the plaques and tangles of AD, plus all the other sources of damage.

Anything you do to promote the overall health of your brain may forestall—or even prevent—memory loss and other AD symptoms.

PROTECT YOUR BRAIN

Many of the same practices that lower your risk for heart attack and stroke also reduce the chances that you will develop AD.

•**Control blood pressure.** High blood pressure can contribute to the narrowing of blood vessels and reduces blood flow to the brain, depriving it of oxygen and nutrients. This makes brain cells more vulnerable to AD damage and raises the risk for ministrokes.

Scientific evidence: Numerous studies have linked increasing blood pressure with declining memory. A Scandinavian study of 1,449 middle-aged volunteers, reported in the *British Medical Journal,* found that those with mild hypertension—130 to 140 systolic (top number)—had twice the chance of having AD 20 years later. Those who had more severe hypertension—141 to 160 systolic—had nearly three times the risk.

Self-defense: Keep your blood pressure at 115/75 or less. If it exceeds 130/90 despite your efforts to bring it down—losing weight, exercising and quitting smoking—you may need medication, such as diuretics, beta-blockers or calcium channel blockers.

•**Lower cholesterol.** High cholesterol levels cause narrowing of blood vessels, which impairs circulation in the brain and may lead to ministrokes. Some research suggests that high cholesterol promotes the development of AD plaques.

Scientific evidence: The same Scandinavian study found that people with total cholesterol above 250 mg/dL were more than twice as likely to develop AD in later life than those with normal levels.

Self-defense: Aim for total cholesterol under 150 mg/dL. A healthy diet, exercise and smoking cessation can help bring it down. If your cholesterol remains above 150, talk to your doctor about medication.

Statins, such as *pravastatin* (Pravachol) and *atorvastatin* (Lipitor), are the drugs of choice for elevated cholesterol. Several studies have found that individuals taking these drugs have 60% to 80% less risk of developing AD than those not taking them.

DIET FOR A HEALTHY BRAIN

Like the rest of your body, your brain must be well fed to function optimally and stay healthy.

•**Eat at least five servings of fruits and vegetables daily.** They contain antioxidant vitamins and phytochemicals that protect brain cells from damage by free radicals.

The best antioxidant food sources: Blueberries, pomegranates, carrots and green, leafy vegetables.

One antioxidant that deserves particular attention is vitamin E.

Scientific evidence: A Dutch study of 5,395 people, age 55 or older, published in the *Journal of the American Medical Association,* found that those consuming the most vitamin E in foods and supplements had 43% less chance of developing AD than those consuming the least.

Increase your intake of vitamin E–rich foods, such as whole grains, avocados and olive oil.

•**Have fish twice weekly.** Cold-water fish, including wild salmon and mackerel, contain omega-3 fatty acids that function as antioxidants as well as counter inflammation that can damage brain cells. Fish consumption also has been linked to improved circulation.

Scientific evidence: A study of 815 people, ages 65 to 94, found that those who consumed fish once or more weekly had 60% less risk of developing AD than those who did not.

•**Drink in moderation.** Temperate consumption of alcohol—two glasses of wine, two beers or one drink containing hard liquor daily—keeps brain cell membranes more flexible, which lets them function better.

Caution: Consuming greater amounts of alcohol, especially as you grow older, has been shown to impair memory and damage brain and other tissues.

Scientific evidence: A Dutch study published in *The Lancet* found that older adults who consumed mild to moderate amounts of alcohol daily had a 42% lower risk for dementia.

ACTIVITY FOR THE BRAIN

Brain function has been shown to improve in people who are active—both mentally and physically.

•**Stay mentally active.** Mental workouts stimulate the release of growth factors—chemicals that spur brain cells to forge a rich network of cells that can compensate if some cells are disabled by AD.

Scientific evidence: A study of 801 Catholic priests and nuns, age 65 or older, found that those who spent the most leisure time in activities that demanded thinking—reading books, playing cards, solving crossword puzzles—had half the AD risk of those who spent the least time involved in such pursuits.

Self-defense: Read books that make you think…follow political developments around the world…learn a foreign language…play games, such as chess, that require cognitive skills.

• **Get regular exercise.** Physical activity stimulates brain growth factors, improves circulation and reduces the risk for ministrokes.

Scientific evidence: A University of California at Los Angeles study that followed 6,000 women, age 65 or older, for six to eight years found that the more miles they walked daily, the lower their risk for dementia. Other studies that included men had similar results.

Self-defense: Just a little exercise makes a lot of difference. Do something active—brisk walking, tennis or dancing—for at least 30 minutes each day.

The Truth About Brain Food

Mark A. Stengler, ND, naturopathic physician…director, La Jolla Whole Health Clinic, La Jolla, CA…adjunct associate clinical professor, National College of Natural Medicine, Portland, OR…author of *The Natural Physician's Healing Therapies* and coauthor of *Prescription for Natural Cures* (both from Bottom Line Books)…and author of the *Bottom Line/Natural Healing* newsletter.

Everyone forgets something from time to time. Some people have trouble remembering names. Others can't keep track of their car keys. Whether we suffer everyday absentmindedness or moments of real memory loss, all of us are concerned about keeping our brain power intact.

In recent years, a great deal of research has focused on the most severe kinds of memory loss—senile dementia and Alzheimer's disease. In the US, these closely related conditions affect up to 10% of people over age 65 and nearly half of those over age 85.

Many studies have identified ways to lower the risk of these age-related problems. Popular methods include stress-reduction strategies, such as daily exercise, positive mental imagery, biofeedback and close personal relationships, to prevent spikes in the memory-draining stress hormone *cortisol*…"brain workouts," including crossword puzzles, word games and challenging card games…and eight to nine hours of sleep each night. Good nutrition—and the right kind of supplementation—also can help protect our brains and safeguard our memories at any age. The sooner you get started with a brain-protecting regimen, the more you'll benefit.

For optimal brain function, your diet should be well-balanced with carbohydrates (40%), protein (30%) and fats (30%). You can accomplish this by eating meals that include whole grains, fruits and vegetables (to get complex carbohydrates)…fish, poultry, lean meats, legumes, nuts and seeds (for protein)…and fish oil, olive oil, avocados, almonds, walnuts and ground flaxseed (for fats). Steer clear of dairy products and packaged and processed foods, such as cookies, white bread and pasta, which are packed with simple carbohydrates that wreak havoc on glucose levels, contributing to diabetes, stroke/vascular disease and dementia.

THE VALUE OF FISH

Fish provides *docosahexaenoic acid* (DHA) and *eicosapentaenoic acid* (EPA), the most plentiful fatty acids in the brain. DHA, an omega-3 fatty acid, is found in abundance in cold-water fish such as mackerel, sardines, salmon and herring. You also can get it from fish-oil supplements, egg yolks, DHA-enriched eggs and some algae supplements, such as Neuromins, a product that is available at most health-food stores.

Foods such as walnuts…leafy, green vegetables…and supplements including flaxseed and hemp oil contain *alpha-linolenic acid,* an omega-3 fatty acid that can be converted by the body into DHA and EPA.

How essential is DHA to memory? It has been known for some years that people have a higher risk of Alzheimer's if they have low blood levels of

DHA. A study in *Archives of Neurology* revealed that people who ate fish one to three times a month had a 40% lower risk of Alzheimer's than those who never ate fish. Those who consumed fish once a week or more had a 60% lower risk. Fish may be baked, broiled or grilled.

It also makes sense to take a fish-oil supplement daily. I suggest 1,000 milligrams (mg) of combined DHA and EPA. Good brands are Nordic Naturals (800-662-2544, *www.nordicnaturals.com*) and Carlson Laboratories (888-234-5656, *www.carlsonlabs.com*), both available at health-food stores.

Caution: Fish oil can thin blood, so check with your physician before using it if you take any blood-thinning medications such as *warfarin* (Coumadin).

GLA IS ESSENTIAL

Omega-6s make up another class of essential fatty acids that are necessary for good brain function. Omega-6 is found in vegetable oils, including safflower, sunflower and corn oils. Most American diets contain too much of these oils due to consumption of packaged and fried foods. However, the most important omega-6 fatty acid is *linoleic acid,* which is converted in the body to *gamma-linolenic acid* (GLA). This essential fatty acid plays a big role in the formation of healthy brain-cell membranes, the part of the cell that stores information. Taking borage oil or evening primrose oil are healthful ways to increase GLA intake—hempseed and hempseed oil also are good sources. Another way to get GLA in the diet is by consuming flaxseed (with water to prevent constipation) or flaxseed oil.

COUNT ON CHOLINE

Just as a car needs spark plugs, an active brain needs quick-firing neurotransmitters. As the name implies, a neurotransmitter sends a signal—one that jumps from one brain cell to another. Substances that act as neurotransmitters —the most important of which is a brain chemical called *acetylcholine*—are vital components of the brain's communication system.

There's one hitch. In order for your body to manufacture enough *acetylcholine,* you need to get a closely related nutrient called *choline.* The best source of choline is *phosphatidylcholine* (PC), which occurs naturally in fish, egg yolks, legumes, nuts, meat and vegetables. It also is found in breast milk. To help prevent memory problems, you can boost your PC intake by taking a 1,500- to 2,000-milligram (mg) PC supplement daily. (Doses of more than 3,000 mg can cause digestive upset, including diarrhea, nausea and stomachache.)

PC is only part of the neurotransmitter equation. To turn PC into brain-friendly *choline,* you also need to get healthy doses of vitamin C and certain B vitamins. You can get plenty of these vitamins in your diet by eating red, yellow and green peppers, citrus fruits and cantaloupe for vitamin C and sweet potatoes, tuna and avocados for B vitamins. Also, I recommend taking a balanced daily multivitamin/mineral supplement.

Deficiencies of folic acid and other key B vitamins have been associated with an increased risk of Alzheimer's disease. These nutrients help to lower levels of *homocysteine,* a harmful by-product of protein metabolism that is increased in people who are genetically susceptible. That's why it is important to have your blood levels of homocysteine, folic acid and B-12 tested by your doctor to see if you need additional supplementation of folic acid and/or B-12.

THE EUROPEAN CURE

For years, European doctors have recommended the supplement called *L-alpha-glycerylphosphorylcholine* (GPC) to promote mental acuity (the ability to respond quickly and appropriately to mental challenges). GPC actually is used by the brain more effectively than PC to form *acetylcholine*—but it costs twice as much and is less widely available in the US. A good GPC supplement by Source Naturals is sold in some health-food stores under the brand name Alpha GPC. Take two 300-mg capsules twice daily for the first four weeks, then two 300-mg capsules once daily as a maintenance dosage. Side effects are rare, but take GPC with a meal if it seems to interfere with your digestion.

PS: BE SURE TO GET MORE

Phosphatidylserine (PS) is a fat that the brain requires to preserve the key brain chemicals *serotonin* and *dopamine.* It also has been shown to reduce levels of the stress hormone cortisol. PS is found in fish, soy and leafy, green vegetables. As we age, PS levels in the body start to decline, so most people need to take a supplement once they're past age 50.

A normal daily diet has about 70 mg of PS. You need about four times that much if you have memory problems. Nearly anyone can benefit from a 300-mg daily supplement of PS. You're likely to notice improvements in mental alertness after four to eight weeks. A small percentage of people have digestive upset, such as bloating and diarrhea, but you can reduce the dosage if this is a problem. PS is available at health-food stores and pharmacies. Make sure you buy a product that lists "phosphatidylserine" on the label. (Some supplements contain "phosphorylated serine," a nutrient complex that doesn't provide the same benefits as PS.) A high-quality PS supplement is made by Jarrow Formulas (to find a retailer, call 800-726-0886 or go to *www.jarrow.com*).

HELP FROM ALC

When taken as a supplement, a nutrient known as *acetyl-L-carnitine* (ALC) has been shown to improve cognitive function and memory in older adults. Researchers also have found that ALC slows the progression of early-stage Alzheimer's disease. By improving communication between the two main hemispheres of the brain, ALC helps enhance the interplay of creative and cognitive brain activity.

For people with mild memory problems, I recommend taking 500 mg of ALC daily on an empty stomach. For those with more severe problems such as dementia, I suggest the same dose three times daily. Cut back if you have digestive upset. Most health-food stores carry a reliable ALC formula produced by Now Foods (888-301-1336, *www.thecatalog.com*).

ADD ANTIOXIDANTS

In all likelihood, Alzheimer's disease and the other types of dementia are related to excessive damage by free radicals (normal by-products of metabolism that can destroy cells, organs and tissues). Free radicals irreversibly injure our cells and contribute to accelerated aging, but studies have shown that this damage can be warded off by getting enough antioxidant nutrients to help guard our brain-cell membranes.

There's ample evidence that a daily dose of 2,000 international units (IU) of the powerful antioxidant vitamin E can slow the decline of cognitive function in people who have moderate to severe Alzheimer's disease. There have been controversial vitamin E studies that seemed to show a link to worsening chronic disease. However, I don't have much confidence in those studies because they were performed on unhealthy people. When it comes to Alzheimer's, results of vitamin E studies have been quite good.

All fresh fruits, vegetables and other plant foods provide multiple naturally occurring antioxidants. Juices are an especially concentrated source of antioxidants. In fact, a study of nearly 2,000 Japanese Americans found that those who reported drinking fruit and vegetable juices at least three times a week had a 75% lower risk of developing dementia than those who drank juices less than once a week. The most nutritious fruit juices include cranberry, pomegranate, apple and blueberry. I also like mixed vegetable juices containing any combination of spinach, celery, lettuce, parsley, watercress, carrot and tomato.

If there is a strong family history of dementia or you have beginning signs of it, take up to 2,000 IU of vitamin E daily.* Green tea also is an excellent source of antioxidants. I recommend drinking two to four cups of green tea daily and eight ounces of fresh juice.

GINKGO—THE BRAIN PLEASER

Ginkgo biloba is an herbal remedy that has been shown to improve memory and cognitive processing by promoting blood flow to the brain. I recommend a 24% *flavoglycoside* extract. Start with a dose of 120 mg to 240 mg daily, and increase to 360 mg daily over a four-week period. Some people begin to see results in four to eight weeks. If you're already taking a blood-thinning medication such as aspirin or *warfarin,* consult your doctor before taking ginkgo.

*Due to the possible interactions between vitamin E and various drugs and supplements as well as other safety considerations, be sure to talk to your doctor before taking vitamin E.

Common Drugs Fight Alzheimer's

Nonsteroidal anti-inflammatory drugs such as *ibuprofen* and *naproxen* seem to help dissolve the brain lesions that occur in Alzheimer's patients, which are caused by plaque buildup. The drugs bond to and help dissolve the plaque, which also prevents new lesions from forming. This suggests that anti-inflammatories may be useful in lowering a person's risk of developing Alzheimer's, but more research is needed.

Gary Small, MD, PhD, director of the University of California at Los Angeles' Center on Aging.

Natural Healers

Shari Lieberman, PhD, a nutrition scientist in Hillsboro Beach, FL, who has been in practice for more than 25 years.

Most health-conscious people do their best to eat plenty of fruits and vegetables. But that's not enough.

Problem: Few people consider the nutrients that are lost after produce is harvested. For example, green vegetables lose almost all of their vitamin C after just a few days of storage at room temperature. What's more, cooking can deplete up to 50% of a variety of vitamins.

Solution: Many doctors now recommend vitamin and mineral supplements to compensate for dietary deficiencies and help prevent chronic diseases, such as heart disease, macular degeneration and osteoarthritis.

Everyone should take a daily multivitamin that provides all of the essential minerals and B vitamins, along with antioxidants, such as vitamins C and E.

Good brands: Solgar and Enzymatic Therapy. Unfortunately, once-a-day supplements provide only *minimal* levels of some important nutrients.

If you have—or are at risk for—one or more of the conditions listed below, you may benefit from taking, in addition to your multivitamin, the following supplements in higher-than-normal "therapeutic" doses.*

DEMENTIA/MEMORY LOSS

Millions of Americans age 65 or older suffer from Alzheimer's disease or age-related memory loss. Many of these older adults are deficient in B vitamins, especially B-12.

*Supplement doses listed here are higher than the recommended daily intake. Because such doses may have unwanted effects, check with your doctor before trying any of these regimens. In rare cases, they may interfere with standard drug treatment.

Key supplements…

• **B-complex supplement** provides the full complement of B vitamins, including B-1, B-2, B-3, B-6 and B-12.

Typical daily therapeutic dose: 50 to 100 milligrams (mg) of B-complex…plus 500 to 1,000 micrograms (mcg) of B-12 in a separate supplement.

• **Alpha-lipoic acid** improves brain function by slowing or stopping the death of nerve cells.

Typical daily therapeutic dose: 600 mg.

• **Vitamin E** protects brain cells from damage caused by disease-causing molecules known as free radicals.

Typical daily therapeutic dose: 1,200 international units (IU).**

• **Ginkgo biloba** improves brain circulation, reduces free-radical damage and may slow the onset of Alzheimer's.

Typical daily therapeutic dose: 240 mg.

Warning: If you are taking a blood-thinning medication, such as *warfarin* (Coumadin), consult your doctor before taking vitamin E or ginkgo biloba. Both have a mild blood-thinning effect.

HEART DISEASE

The standard drugs—such as nitroglycerin for treating angina and statins for lowering cholesterol—mainly manage heart disease symptoms, not the underlying causes. Statins lower levels of harmful LDL cholesterol, but they also deplete coenzyme Q10 (CoQ10) from heart cells. This naturally occurring enzyme is believed to strengthen the heart muscle.

Key supplements…

• **CoQ10.** All people with heart disease should ask their cardiologist about taking it. Studies have demonstrated that CoQ10 improves symptoms associated with congestive heart failure, angina and other heart disorders. In some cases, people who take the enzyme are even able to reduce their doses of heart medications.

Typical daily therapeutic dose: 50 to 300 mg. Start with the lower dose and gradually increase it until you notice a reduction of symptoms. Do *not* stop taking CoQ10 abruptly. Doing so can cause a rebound of symptoms.

**Choose natural vitamin E (d-alpha tocopherol), which is more effective than the synthetic version.

• **Fish oil** lowers levels of C-reactive protein, a "marker" for artery inflammation that accompanies heart disease.

Typical daily therapeutic dose: 3 to 6 grams (g).

Helpful: Enteric-coated fish oil capsules dissolve in the intestine and are less likely than other products to cause a fishy taste when you burp.

Warning: Fish oil capsules can have a blood-thinning effect.

• **Antioxidant supplements** prevent cell damage in artery walls and reduce inflammation.

Typical daily therapeutic dose: 400 to 1,200 IU vitamin E…1 to 4 g vitamin C…and 25,000 IU natural beta-carotene.

• **Niacin** works as well as some statins at lowering total cholesterol—and it increases levels of beneficial HDL cholesterol. Combining niacin with a statin may allow you to take a lower dose of the statin drug. Because niacin can cause flushing, look for a "flush-free" product. At high doses, niacin can also cause liver problems, so use it only under a doctor's supervision.

Typical daily therapeutic dose: 2 g.

MACULAR DEGENERATION

Macular degeneration is caused by a breakdown of the *macula,* the part of the retina that is responsible for central vision. It's the main cause of severe vision loss in people age 50 or older. *Key supplements…*

• **Carotenoids,** especially beta-carotene and lutein, are used by the eye to build and repair damaged cells.

Typical daily therapeutic dose: 25,000 IU natural beta-carotene and 10 to 15 mg lutein.

• **Vitamin E** reduces oxidative stress in the eye and prevents further damage.

Typical daily therapeutic dose: 800 IU.

• **Zinc** is used by the eye to manufacture chemical compounds that aid vision.

Typical daily therapeutic dose: 22 to 50 mg.

OSTEOARTHRITIS

Osteoarthritis is the most common form of arthritis and the leading cause of pain and disability in older Americans. The anti-inflammatory analgesics, such as *ibuprofen* (Advil), are effective but often cause side effects, such as gastrointestinal bleeding.

Key supplements…

• **Fish oil** reduces levels of *arachidonic acid,* a fatty acid that forms inflammatory, joint-damaging chemicals known as prostaglandins.

Typical daily therapeutic dose: 3 to 6 g.

• **Vitamins C and E** block the effects of inflammatory free radicals in the joints. They work synergistically with fish oil to enhance its effects.

Typical daily therapeutic dose: 4 g vitamin C…and 400 to 1,200 IU vitamin E.

• **Quercetin,** a plant-based flavonoid, relieves pain as well as ibuprofen does.

Typical daily therapeutic dose: 2 to 4 g.

The Oxygen Cure

Daniel Hamner, MD, sports medicine physician and owner and founder of the Peak Energy Program in New York City. He is coauthor of *Peak Energy: The High-Oxygen Program for More Energy Now.* St. Martin's.

Every cell in the body requires oxygen to function properly. The brain alone uses at least 12% of the total oxygen that people inhale.

Problem: The breathing habits of most people *don't* always provide all the oxygen that the brain and body need.

Oxygen deprivation is a leading cause of persistent fatigue—a condition that accounts for up to 15 million doctor visits annually, making it one of the most common health problems in the US. It also causes mental fogginess and, in some cases, depression.

My story: For years, I barely had enough energy to get through my workdays. I started reading about energy-building techniques—everything from yoga to the latest research in exercise physiology. I quickly realized that all of these techniques aim to increase oxygen levels in the body.

At the age of 47, I developed—and began practicing—a high-oxygen program. Within a matter of months, my oxygen usage rose from 42.7 milliliters of oxygen per kilogram of body weight per minute up to 55 milliliters—a 30%

increase. At the same time, my energy levels rose dramatically.

7 STEPS TO BETTER OXYGENATION

Nearly everyone can increase oxygen levels and experience a significant boost in energy in as little as two weeks. *Here's how…*

•*Step 1:* **Take a pro-oxygenator.** The herbal supplement ginseng enhances the body's ability to utilize oxygen. A four-week study of oxygen utilization found that people taking ginseng experienced a 29% improvement in oxygen transportation to tissues and organs.

Typical dose: 400 to 600 milligrams (mg) once daily.

Caution: Do not take ginseng if you have high blood pressure. If you are taking medication, consult your physician before trying ginseng.

•*Step 2:* **Stand up straight.** Poor posture—rounding the shoulders, stooping forward, etc.—can inhibit oxygen intake.

People who stand straight, roll back their shoulders, push their chests out while squeezing their shoulder blades together and keep their chin up can increase lung capacity by 5%.

Helpful: To ensure proper form, practice this while looking in a full-length mirror.

•*Step 3:* **Exercise.** Aerobic exercise increases pathways in the body that carry oxygen to cells. People who start an aerobic exercise program experience an immediate increase in oxygen usage and energy.

My recommendation: Walk fast, run, swim, bike, etc.—for a minimum of 60 minutes three days a week.

Resistance training increases strength and endurance. Consult a physical trainer or other exercise professional for a strength-training regimen that works the muscles in your upper and lower body and your core (trunk).

My recommendation: Twenty to 30 minutes of strength training at least three times a week.

•*Step 4:* **Eat "charge-up" foods.** A diet high in complex carbohydrates—fruits (such as apples and oranges)…vegetables (such as carrots and spinach)…whole grains…legumes (such as black beans)…etc.—significantly improves the blood's ability to transport oxygen to cells. A high-fat diet does the opposite—it reduces the blood's oxygen-carrying capacity.

•*Step 5:* **Practice instant-energy breathing.** You can reverse fatigue almost instantly with a yoga breathing technique that floods cells with oxygen and boosts energy for 15 minutes or more. *What to do…*

•Sit up straight and take 20 to 30 quick, panting breaths. Only your belly should move, not your chest.

•Take a deep breath, filling your lungs with air…and hold for 30 seconds. If you can, gradually work up to holding your breath for 60 seconds.

•Exhale completely. Press your hand down against your belly. This puts pressure on your lungs and forces out more of the used air.

After completing the exercise, walk briskly for 10 minutes, if possible. This will pull additional air into your lungs and increase the circulation of oxygen-rich blood cells.

•*Step 6:* **Stop smoking—and avoid secondhand smoke.** Smokers tend to have less energy and more depression than nonsmokers, in part because they get less blood and oxygen to the brain. Smoking—as well as exposure to secondhand smoke—increases blood levels of carbon monoxide, a waste chemical that increases fatigue. It also causes higher levels of arterial plaque—fatty accumulations that inhibit circulation.

Smokers who attend smoking cessation programs, such as SmokEnders, or use stop-smoking products, such as nicotine patches, are about twice as likely to quit the habit as those who try to stop on their own.

Important: Take 1,000 mg of vitamin C daily when trying to quit smoking. Each cigarette inactivates 25 mg of vitamin C in the body.

•*Step 7:* **See a doctor if you have low energy.** Fatigue is a common first symptom of hundreds of medical conditions, including iron-deficiency anemia, food allergies, heart problems and cancer. Consult your doctor if you experience mental fogginess or low physical energy for more than a few weeks.

ARE YOU GETTING ENOUGH OXYGEN?

Most people can check their own oxygen levels with this simple test…

•**Stand in front of a step.** Relax for a moment, then check your resting heart rate.

To do this: Place the tips of your index and middle fingers on the thumb side of your wrist. Count your heartbeats for 30 seconds, then multiply by two.

● **Rapidly step onto and off of the step for one minute.** Check your heart rate again. It probably has risen quite a bit—from, say, 80 beats to 120 beats per minute.

● **Rest for one minute, then check your heart rate again.** If it returned to the resting level, your blood is carrying adequate oxygen. If it stayed elevated above the resting level for more than one minute, your heart is trying to compensate for low blood levels of oxygen.

Vibrant Health via Nutraceuticals

Mary E. O'Brien, MD, a board-certified internist in Myrtle Beach, SC. She is cochair of the medical advisory board of the American Nutraceutical Association, *www. ana-jana.org,* and coeditor of *Nutraceuticals: The Complete Encyclopedia of Supplements, Herbs, Vitamins and Healing Foods.* Perigee.

Echinacea, St. John's wort and other supplements have become big sellers in this country. But most Americans have yet to discover the full array of herbs, vitamins and minerals that can be used to relieve—or prevent—many health conditions.

Known as *nutraceuticals,** these supplements are derived from—or, in some cases, mimic—chemically active compounds found in plants.

Unlike over-the-counter or prescription drugs, which typically treat specific symptoms, some nutraceuticals may reduce oxidative damage by free radicals, which can contribute to heart disease and other chronic conditions. For some ailments, they can be just as effective as drugs but usually cause fewer side effects and cost less. Ask your doctor which products might be appropriate for you.

*The US Food and Drug Administration (FDA) does not regulate supplements or herbs. Always check with your doctor before taking any of these products. They can interact with prescription medications.

FATIGUE
A century ago, the average American slept 10 hours a night. Now the average American gets only seven hours of sleep each night. *To curb fatigue, try...*

● **Coenzyme Q10 (CoQ10)**—30 milligrams (mg) twice daily. It plays a crucial role in the production of *adenosine triphosphate* (ATP), a molecule that is used throughout the body as a source of energy.

Helpful: Combine CoQ10 with 60 mg of the amino acid *carnitine* twice daily. This regimen activates energy-producing components (mitochondria) inside cells, which may boost energy and stamina.

● **Ginseng**—Begin with 100 mg once a day. The dose can be gradually increased up to 300 mg twice daily. Ginseng may function as a mild stimulant and has been used in Asian cultures to increase stamina and enhance well-being.

Caution: Ginseng can be harmful for people with high blood pressure, angina, headaches or hyperthyroidism.

HIGH BLOOD PRESSURE
Several of my patients have tried as many as four blood pressure drugs without being able to control their condition. *Ensuring adequate levels of certain nutrients may improve blood pressure control...*

● **Essential fatty acids (EFAs)**—Found in salmon and other cold-water fish, flaxseed, walnuts and other nuts, EFAs may help prevent arterial damage caused by high blood pressure. Sprinkle flaxseed on salads and cereals. Eat cold-water fish at least twice a week.

● **Magnesium**—750 mg daily. It helps regulate the relaxation and constriction of blood vessels. This may lower blood pressure.

● **Potassium**—2,000 mg daily. It is essential in regulating heartbeat. It can also lower systolic pressure (upper number) by four points and diastolic pressure (lower number) by three points, according to a recent study.

Caution: Limit supplemental potassium to 500 mg daily. Get the remainder of your daily intake from potassium-rich foods—apricots, bananas, cantaloupe, potatoes and spinach.

MEMORY PROBLEMS

• **Docosahexanoic acid (DHA)**—3 to 6 g daily. DHA is the most abundant fatty acid in the brain, but the modern diet may not provide enough. Foods that are rich in DHA include eggs, organ meats, cold-water fish and wild game.

• **Folate**—800 micrograms (mcg) daily. It lowers levels of the blood protein *homocysteine,* reducing the risk for stroke and other vascular events that can lead to dementia. Recent research suggests that low levels of folate may be linked to Alzheimer's disease.

• **Ginkgo**—60 mg twice daily. It increases blood flow to parts of the brain that lack sufficient circulation. It has no effect when blood flow is normal.

Caution: Ginkgo interferes with blood clotting. It should *not* be used by people taking non-steroidal anti-inflammatory drugs (NSAIDs), such as aspirin, ibuprofen, etc., or prescription blood thinners, such as *warfarin* (Coumadin).

• **Vitamin E**—100 to 400 international units (IU) daily.* This antioxidant blocks the oxidation of LDL (bad) cholesterol and may slow the progression of Alzheimer's disease.

OSTEOARTHRITIS

It's been called "wear-and-tear" arthritis—but research suggests that the disorder results from poor cartilage regeneration. *To curb osteoarthritis, try...*

• **Glucosamine**—500 mg three times daily. It may improve cartilage thickness and help repair existing damage. For many people, pain relief begins in four weeks.

• **Vitamin C**—100 mg twice daily. The Framingham Heart Study showed that vitamin C can slow the progression of pain due to osteoarthritis of the knee.

PROSTATE ENLARGEMENT

More than half of men age 60 and older suffer from prostate enlargement. Benign prostatic hypertrophy (BPH) can result in urinary frequency, irritation or difficulty urinating. *To curb symptoms of prostate enlargement, try...*

*Due to the possible interactions between vitamin E and various drugs and supplements as well as other safety considerations, be sure to talk to your doctor before taking vitamin E.

• **Pygeum africanum**—100 to 200 mg daily. This African herb contains *pentacyclic triterpenes,* chemicals that shrink prostate tissue. It also reduces prostate irritation.

• **Saw palmetto**—60 mg twice daily. It may reduce prostate irritation within four weeks. *Finasteride* (Proscar), a prescription drug often prescribed for BPH, generally takes up to four months to work.

Caution: Taking saw palmetto may mask a high prostate-specific antigen (PSA) level. Before taking saw palmetto, see your doctor for a baseline PSA test.

• **Zinc**—15 to 30 mg per day. It is important for normal prostate health and boosts immune function.

Good sources from foods: Pumpkin seeds, red meat, shellfish, oysters, nuts and wheat germ.

Scents to Boost Energy, Mood, Memory and More

Alan R. Hirsch, MD, founder and neurological director of the Smell & Taste Treatment and Research Foundation in Chicago. He is a neurologist and psychiatrist, and author of *Life's a Smelling Success* (Authors of Unity) and *What Flavor Is Your Personality?* (Sourcebooks).

Scents stimulate important mental and physical functions. They trigger the release of neurotransmitters, chemicals that send signals to the brain. *Here is a sampling of what scents can do for you...*

CONTROL APPETITE

In a study of 105 people, we found that those who inhaled a chocolate-like aroma whenever they felt like eating lost nearly three pounds in two weeks. One study of 3,193 volunteers found that sniffing banana, green apple or peppermint scents resulted in an average weight loss of 30 pounds in six months.

Sniff the above scents often, and remember to smell every food before you eat it. Your brain will perceive that you're eating more, thus suppressing your appetite.

INCREASE ENERGY

These odors stimulate the part of the brain that promotes wakefulness...

- **Jasmine** causes an increase in beta waves in the brain, a sign of alertness. Jasmine tea is a great pick-me-up.

- **Strawberries** and buttered popcorn will cause exercisers to burn more calories.

- **Peppermint** works on sensory nerves and increases alertness. Try a peppermint candy or chewing gum.

- **Freshly brewed coffee** is very stimulating, probably because we associate the aroma with the energizing effects of caffeine.

BOOST ROMANCE

Both men and women are sexually stimulated by scents, but the odors that arouse them aren't the same.

For men: The smell of lavender or pumpkin pie increases blood flow to the penis by about 40%. The smell of doughnuts, black licorice, vanilla or women's perfume (any scent) also is sexually stimulating to men.

For women: The odors of cucumber and licorice are stimulating. Women are turned off by the smells of cherries, barbecued meat and men's cologne.

REDUCE ANXIETY

Fresh, natural scents, in general, induce calm. In one study we conducted, volunteers became extremely anxious when they were confined in coffin-like tubes, but then calmed down when the tubes were infused with the smells of green apple and cucumber. These odors seem to have an impact on the limbic system, the emotional center of the brain.

If you anticipate a situation in which you will feel anxious, wash your hair that morning with a green-apple–scented shampoo and/or put a dab of the shampoo in a cloth to take with you.

IMPROVE MEMORY

People who sniff floral scents increase retention of new material by 17%.

Sniff a floral odor when learning new material, then smell it again when you want to recall it. This is known as *state-dependent learning.* The material you learn in one state—while smelling roses—will be more accessible when you replicate that state in the future.

Herbs That Boost Your Immunity

Kathy Abascal, RH, a registered herbalist with the American Herbalists Guild who practices herbal medicine in Vashon, Washington. She is the author of *Herbs & Influenza: How Herbs Used in the 1918 Flu Pandemic Can Be Effective Today.* Tigana.

While scientists are furiously working to develop a vaccine and/or a drug treatment to help protect us against the world's next major outbreak of influenza, many herbalists believe that potentially effective natural medicines already exist.

Within the last century, three influenza pandemics—in 1918, 1957 and 1968—killed millions of people worldwide. Medical science has changed dramatically since the outbreaks, but a little-known yet highly effective approach to treating the flu of 1918 may prevent people from contracting the illness during a future outbreak—or help aid in recovery if they do become sick.

NEW LESSONS FROM OLD RESEARCH

In 1918 and 1919, a strain of influenza dubbed "the Spanish flu" (in part because it received the most press coverage in Spain, which was not preoccupied with World War I) circled the globe and resulted in not just one, but two (and in some places three) waves of deadly illness. The Spanish flu and its associated complications, including pneumonia and pleurisy (inflammation of the covering of the lungs), killed as many as 50 million people worldwide.

Some people received what were then believed to be the most progressive and scientific conventional treatments available—mercury, strong laxatives, aspirin, arsenic, quinine and a mixture of ipecac and opium called Dover's powder. According to the Centers for Disease Control and Prevention, more than 2.5%, or 25 out of every 1,000 people treated conventionally, died.

Surveys from the period show that patients given herbal remedies used by a nationwide group of physicians who called themselves the "Eclectics"—because they practiced "eclectic" medicine (what we today might call herbal or alternative medicine)—died at a rate of 0.6%, meaning that six out of every 1,000 who received these botanical treatments died.

Who documented this huge disparity? At the onset of the Spanish flu outbreak, John Lloyd was a respected pharmacist, plant extract researcher, past president of the American Pharmaceutical Association, and an owner, with his brothers, of Lloyd Brothers, a Cincinnati, Ohio–located distributor of pharmaceutical botanicals.

In 1919—when the Spanish flu pandemic was on the wane—Lloyd conducted a survey of 222 physicians who had purchased his company's herbal products, asking which ones they had used to treat influenza and pneumonia, how the products were administered and which of the treatments they considered to be the most effective.

Respondents named more than 40 botanical treatments, including *gelsemium* (the dried root and rhizome of the yellow jasmine plant native to the Southeastern US), *echinacea* (purple coneflowers that are native to Midwestern North America), *aconite* (a bluish flowered herb of the buttercup family) and *boneset* (a white-flowered plant native to Eastern North America).

Most of the Eclectics practiced "specific medication," treating the flu by addressing each individual patient's specific symptoms—respiratory illness, fever, coughs, vomiting, fatigue, etc. This approach differed from that of conventional doctors, who treated every influenza patient basically the same with purgatives, quinine, aspirin and Dover's powder, regardless of the individual's symptoms.

INCREASE YOUR IMMUNITY

A number of herbal medicines can be used to strengthen the immune system.

The herbs listed below are generally safe and are widely available at health-food stores.* Good manufacturers that offer all these herbs include Herbalist & Alchemist (*www.herbalist-alchemist. com*) and Herb Pharm (*www.herb-pharm.com*).

Adaptogens are herbs used to balance the immune system. They work slowly, so they should be started six to eight weeks before the flu season (typically November to April) and continued throughout that period. Also, adaptogens can be used as needed for general immunity strength-

*Check with your health-care provider before using these herbals, especially if you are taking prescription medications, such as blood thinners or drugs to treat high blood pressure or diabetes. Pregnant and nursing women, in particular, should be especially careful to consult a professional before using herbs.

ening to help fight colds and other respiratory ailments.

Take one of the following...

●**Ginseng.** Chinese or Asian ginseng (*Panax ginseng*) and American ginseng (*Panax quinquefolium*) have been used for centuries to fight fatigue and increase immunity. Siberian ginseng, or eleuthero (*Eleutherococcus senticosus*), has similar properties but it is not a member of the ginseng family.

Immune-boosting dosage: Chinese and Asian ginseng: 5 milliliters (ml) to 10 ml of tincture daily...American ginseng: 3 ml to 5 ml of tincture three times daily...Siberian ginseng: 3 ml of tincture three times daily.

●**Ashwagandha** (*Withania somnifera*). Ashwagandha has been used for more than 4,000 years in India to treat and fight infectious diseases and immune system disorders.

Immune-boosting dosage: 3 ml of tincture three times daily.

●**Astragalus** (*Astragalus membranaceus* and related plants). Though little research has been conducted on this herb in the West, it has been used here since the 1800s to strengthen the immune and respiratory systems.

Immune-boosting dosage: 4 ml to 8 ml of tincture three times daily.

THE ECLECTICS' FLU TREATMENT

Herbs used by the Eclectics to treat influenza included echinacea (*Echinacea purpurea, Echinacea angustifolia* and *Echinacea pallida*) and boneset (*Eupatorium perfoliatum*). Echinacea is traditionally utilized to boost immune functioning at the onset of a cold or flu, while boneset is used to reduce fever and relieve aches and pains caused by the flu.

Dosage: For echinacea, mix one ounce of tincture in four ounces of water and take one teaspoon every waking half hour for up to 14 days. For boneset, mix 1 ml to 2 ml in one ounce of warm water and take every one to two waking hours.

USING HERBS SAFELY

The American Herbalists Guild (203-272-6731, *www.americanherbalistsguild.com*) and the American Association of Naturopathic Physicians (866-538-2267, *www.naturopathic.org*) can help you find a qualified practitioner of herbal medicine in your area. Like all medicines, some herbs can be harmful if taken in the wrong quantities or combinations.

Natural Sex Boosters

Ray Sahelian, MD, a board-certified family-practice physician and nutritional consultant in private practice in Marina del Rey, CA. He is author of *Natural Sex Boosters* (Square One) and *Mind-Boosting Secrets* (Bottom Line Books, *www.bottomlinesecrets.com*).

The drug *sildenafil* (Viagra), introduced in 1998, revolutionized the treatment of sexual dysfunction. However, it and related drugs, such as *vardenafil* (Levitra) and *tadalafil* (Cialis), have significant limitations.

Although these impotence medications work well at promoting blood flow to the penis, they have little or no effect on libido or sexual sensation in men—or in women.

These drugs also have potentially serious side effects, such as vision problems, and some doctors believe that they may be dangerous for men who have cardiac conditions, such as irregular heart rhythms, history of heart attack or heart failure.

However, sex-boosting herbs have been used successfully for hundreds of years in Brazil, China, India and parts of Africa.

The following supplements, available at most health-food stores, can improve virtually all aspects of sexual performance, including increased desire, improved genital blood flow in men and women, and stronger erections.*

Start by choosing one herb that seems to best fit your needs. After one to two weeks, you can combine it with another supplement to enhance the effect. Or simply use a formula that combines these herbs.

Important: When combining herbs, cut the recommended dose of each in half to avoid potential side effects, such as restlessness.

HORNY GOAT WEED

This herb increases energy and libido in both men and women...and it may produce firmer erections in men.

*Check with your doctor before taking any of these products.

Horny goat weed reportedly got its name when a Chinese herder noticed that his goats became more sexually active after eating the plant. It's thought to influence levels of *dopamine* and other neurotransmitters that affect libido and mood. It also contains flavonoids, plant chemicals that dilate blood vessels and promote erections.

Scientific evidence: A study conducted in Beijing on 34 patients receiving dialysis for renal failure found that horny goat weed enhanced sexual activity in the patients taking it.

Typical dose: 500 to 2,000 milligrams (mg) daily. Start with 500 mg and increase, if needed. Side effects include restlessness and insomnia.

MUIRA PUAMA

This herb increases libido...orgasm intensity ...and skin and genital sensitivity in men and women.

The bark and roots of this Amazon tree, sometimes known as "potency wood," increase sexual desire and sexual fantasies in men and women, and also facilitate a woman's ability to have an orgasm. It appears to work by promoting blood flow to the genitals in men and women.

Scientific evidence: A clinical study of 262 men, conducted at the Institute of Sexology in Paris, found that taking muira puama for two weeks improved libido in 62% of those studied.

Typical dose: 500 to 1,000 mg in capsule form three consecutive days each week.

Important: Muira puama should be taken in the morning. That's because it can cause insomnia when taken in the afternoon or at night. Muira puama may cause restlessness in some people during the daytime.

TRIBULUS

This herb increases energy and libido in both men and women...and it also improves erections in men.

This common roadside weed contains *protodioscin,* a chemical compound that is thought to increase production of the sex hormone testosterone in both men and women. It also dilates blood vessels in the penis, promoting firmer erections.

Scientific evidence: An animal study conducted at the National University Hospital in Singapore showed that rats that were given tribulus for eight weeks were found to experience firmer erections.

Typical dose: 500 to 1,000 mg daily. Take tribulus for one week, then stop for one week, and so on.

This minimizes the risk for potential side effects, such as restlessness and increased body temperature.

ASHWAGANDHA

This herb increases mood and sexual desire and function in men and women. It can improve sex drive in both sexes by acting as a relaxant. It also assists men in maintaining an erection.

Ashwagandha produces a calming effect by mimicking the action of GABA, a neurotransmitter in the brain that promotes relaxation. It also boosts nitric oxide production. Nitric oxide is known to enhance penile erection and vaginal sensitivity by increasing engorgement of the genital organs through blood vessel dilation.

Scientific evidence: A laboratory study conducted at the University of Texas Health Science Center found that ashwagandha inhibits the number of nerve cells that fire in the brain, much like the neurotransmitter GABA, resulting in an antianxiety and mood-enhancing effect.

Typical dose: 300 to 500 mg one to two times daily.

Important: For better absorption, take ashwagandha on an empty stomach.

Caution: Ashwagandha may cause drowsiness in some individuals. Do not drive after taking this herb.

Alleviate Neck and Back Pain with Fish Oil

When neck and back pain sufferers took a fish-oil supplement (1,200 milligrams [mg] daily) for 75 days, 60% reported significant pain relief that allowed them to decrease or discontinue use of painkillers.

Theory: The omega-3 fatty acids found in fish oil block the inflammation that can lead to neck and back pain. Fish oil also may help relieve joint pain.

If you have neck or back pain: Ask your doctor about taking fish oil. Do not use fish oil if you take *warfarin* (Coumadin) or another blood thinner.

Joseph Maroon, MD, clinical professor of neurological surgery at the University of Pittsburgh School of Medicine and team neurosurgeon to the Pittsburgh Steelers.

Drug-Free Ways To Treat Pain

Norman Marcus, MD, director of the Norman Marcus Pain Institute, New York City. He is clinical associate professor in psychiatry at New York University School of Medicine, and author of *Freedom from Pain.* Fireside.

More than 50 million Americans now suffer from chronic pain—much of it untreated. But when pain sufferers do get medical care, they often receive *overtreatment.* Why is that?

Insurance companies and Medicare reimburse doctors for surgery and other invasive procedures—so that's what doctors are likely to provide. Insurance doesn't pay doctors to counsel patients about low-tech remedies, such as exercise and stress relief—even though these sometimes are the best ways to deal with persistent pain.

Here's how pain problems are frequently misdiagnosed and mistreated—and what you can do to get effective, commonsense pain relief…

BACK PAIN

Up to 80% of Americans suffer from low back pain at some point in their lives. Medical treatment for this chronic problem is based on the assumption that anatomical problems, such as herniated discs, cause the pain. A standard treatment is to operate, sometimes by surgically fusing the vertebrae (bones of the spine).

In reality, bones and discs usually don't cause low back pain. Sprained or strained muscles, ligaments and tendons—soft tissue made vulnerable to injury by overexertion and lack of exercise—underlie most cases.

Scientific evidence: In a study published in *Spine,* orthopedic surgeons treated 64 patients, ages 25 to 60, who had low back pain that had lasted one year or longer. X-rays showed degenerated discs. Half the group received surgery (fusion of the lumbar vertebrae). Half got nonsurgical treatments, including counseling and exercise.

A year after treatment, researchers evaluated both groups for pain, use of pain medication and other factors indicating treatment success or failure. The nonsurgery group had a *higher* success rate—76% compared with 70% of the surgery group (a clinically significant difference). And the nonsurgery group hadn't been subjected to the pain, risk and inconvenience of surgery.

NECK PAIN

In patients over age 40 who suffer from neck pain, a magnetic resonance imaging (MRI) scan or X-ray usually reveals degenerative changes in the vertebrae of the neck. Surgery may be recommended, but these changes are not the cause of most cases of neck pain.

A classic cause of neck (and shoulder) pain is working at a computer where the keyboard is too high or the chair too low—forcing the forearms into a position that creates a less than 90-degree angle in the elbow. This raises shoulder muscles, causing tension and pain in the neck and shoulders. Other common causes of neck pain are reading or watching television in bed and cradling the telephone on your shoulder.

SHOULDER PAIN

Shoulder pain and stiffness frequently are diagnosed as a rotator cuff tear, adhesive capsulitis (frozen shoulder) or "impingement syndrome" (a narrowed amount of space between two rotator cuff muscles).

Your doctor may recommend surgery, followed by painful rehabilitation that might last as long as five months. Pain is generally relieved, but in some cases, patients never regain full function. A nonsurgical treatment to restore strength and flexibility to shoulder muscles can work as well as surgery—and there's no harm in trying it first.

Scientific evidence: Six months after "conservative" treatment for shoulder pain—shoulder exercises, physical therapy, ultrasound and pain-relieving steroid injections—64 out of 82 patients had significant pain relief and increased function,

according to a study published in *Archives of Physical Medicine and Rehabilitation.*

HEADACHE

People with chronic migraine or tension headaches or both (mixed headache syndrome) usually are prescribed pain medications—which are costly and can damage the stomach, liver and/ or kidneys with long-term use. But chronically tense midback, neck and shoulder muscles are a common cause of headache—and muscle tension can be treated without drugs.

Scientific evidence: A study published in *Cochrane Database of Systematic Review*s analyzed 22 other scientific studies on headache treatments, with a total of 2,628 participants. The nondrug therapies, such as spinal manipulation, were as effective as medications—or even more so—for reducing the incidence of migraine or chronic tension headaches.

BETTER WAYS TO REDUCE PAIN

• **Find a pain specialist.** Your first stop should be your primary care physician, who can refer you to a pain specialist. He/she can perform a physical examination that evaluates muscles surrounding the painful joint for strength and flexibility as well as for spasm and trigger points (a tender muscle that refers pain to another part of the body)—an assessment that will show if muscles are causing the pain. If you need help locating a pain specialist, consult the American Academy of Pain Medicine, *www.painmed.org.*

• **Exercise.** Inactivity is the number-one cause of pain. Perform aerobic exercise daily.

Example: Brisk walking—quickly enough to break a sweat—two to three miles a day. Most people who also perform the following exercises daily will notice improvement in the first three weeks, with additional results in six months.*

*These exercises were created by Hans Kraus, MD, former associate professor of clinical physical medicine and rehabilitation at New York University Medical College. Dr. Kraus, who died in 1996, was national chairman of the medical committee for the YMCA's exercise program for back pain and personal physician to former President John F. Kennedy. For a copy of the complete Kraus Exercise Program, visit Dr. Marcus' Web site at *http://backpainusa.com,* or send a self-addressed, stamped envelope to Norman Marcus, MD, "Pain Exercises," 30 E. 40 St., New York, NY 10016.

BEST EXERCISES FOR LOW BACK PAIN

Perform four repetitions of each of the following basic lower-body exercises daily...

1. Diaphragmatic breathing. Lie on your back, arms at your sides and knees bent. Slowly inhale through your nose to make your belly round. Then exhale through your mouth.

2. Shoulder shrug. Pull your shoulders up toward your ears as you inhale through your nose. Then exhale through your mouth as you let your shoulders fall back down.

3. Leg slide. Lie on your back, arms at your sides and knees bent. Slide your right leg down until it is flat on the floor. Relax the right leg for three seconds. Slide your right leg back to bent position. Repeat with your left leg.

4. Head rotation. Lie on your back, arms at your sides and knees bent. Drop your head to the left side. Return your head to center. Then drop your head to the right side.

5. Single knee to chest. Lie on your back, arms at your sides and knees bent. Bring your left knee to your chest as far as you comfortably can. Return your left leg to bent-knee position, then let it slide down until it is flat on the floor. Relax the left leg for three seconds, then slide it back to the bent-knee position. Repeat with your right leg.

6. Side-lying knee to chest. Lie on your left side, knees bent, head resting on your elbow. Bring your right leg toward your chest, letting the knee drop toward the floor. Then slide your right leg back, extending the knee until your leg is straight. Bring your leg back to the starting position. Roll onto your opposite side and repeat.

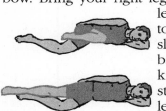

7. Buttocks squeeze. Lie on your stomach and place a pillow under your belly. Tighten your buttocks muscles and hold for two seconds. Relax the muscles.

BEST EXERCISES FOR NECK PAIN, SHOULDER PAIN AND HEADACHE

Perform four repetitions of each of the following basic upper-body exercises daily. Begin with lower-body exercises 1, 2 and 4 (under "Best Exercises for Low Back Pain").

4. Elbow bend. Lie on your back, arms at your sides and legs extended. As you slowly inhale through your nose, close your fists and bend your elbows. Bring both arms toward your head. As you slowly exhale through your mouth, relax your arms and hands and let your arms drop back to your sides.

5. Chicken wings. Lie on your back, arms at your sides and legs extended. Rest your hands on your chest, elbows at your sides. Keeping your elbows down as much as possible, move them so they're pointing behind you. Then return to your starting position.

6. Horizontal abduction–adduction. Lie on your back, hands at your sides and legs extended. Extend your right arm out to the side. Bring your right arm across your chest. Then return it to the extended position. Repeat with your left arm.

7. Shoulder rotation. Lie on your back, arms at your sides and legs extended. Extend your right arm out to the side. Bend your elbow and point your fingers behind you, getting your arm as flat on the floor as possible. Keeping your elbow on the floor, raise your arm 90 degrees so that your fingers are pointing toward the ceiling. Do again. Then move your arm toward the ground, palm down, placing your arm as flat on the floor as possible. Raise your arm 90 degrees, fingers pointing toward the ceiling. Repeat. Perform the entire sequence with your left arm.

8. Shoulder bend. Lie on your back, arms at your sides and legs extended. As you slowly inhale through your nose, extend your arms behind your head, arms as flat on the floor as possible. As you slowly exhale out through your mouth, return your arms to the starting position.

Illustrations by Shawn Banner.

Duct Tape Really Can Cure Warts

Placing duct tape (or other tape) over warts to get rid of them is not just an old wives' tale. A recent study found that placing tape over warts is more effective at eliminating them than standard medical therapy.

The study: Participants who had warts on fingers, palms, heels or soles of the feet were divided into two groups. One group put tape on warts for six days, then soaked the warts and scraped them with emery boards, waited 12 hours and reapplied the tape, repeating the process. The other group had their warts frozen off by a doctor, which is standard therapy.

Result: After just two months, 85% of those using the tape had gotten rid of their warts, versus only 60% of those who had received the standard freezing treatment.

Dean R. Focht III, MD, fellow, division of gastroenterology, hepatology and nutrition, Cincinnati Children's Hospital Medical Center.

Mighty Matcha

The type of green tea used in Japanese tea ceremonies provides 200 times more *epigallocatechin gallate,* a potent anticancer chemical, than the green tea that's served in the US. Known as matcha, the Japanese tea is powdered before steeping—a technique that is believed to release more of the active compound than crumpled leaves. Matcha is available in some health-food stores and on the Web at *www.stashtea.com.*

Science News, 1719 N St. NW, Washington, DC 20036.

Amazing! Salsa Stops Disease

Isao Kubo, PhD, professor, department of nutritional science and toxicology, University of California, Berkeley.

Salsa is not only a favorite tasty food, but it turns out to be a healthy one, too. It can actually *protect* and prevent you from getting sick. Cilantro, one of the common ingredients in this popular Mexican condiment, contains a compound that kills *Salmonella* bacteria, a frequent and sometimes lethal cause of food-borne illness, according to results of a study reported in the *Journal of Agricultural and Food Chemistry.*

EAT YOUR SALSA

Isao Kubo, PhD, lead researcher at the University of California, Berkeley, says that *dodecenal*—a compound that can be isolated from cilantro leaves—is the key Salmonella killer. Researchers were surprised to learn that dodecenal is the only natural antibacterial agent thus far known to be more effective than *gentamicin,* a powerful antibiotic medication that used to be prescribed by doctors to combat Salmonella.

In fact, in laboratory research, dodecenal has proved to be twice as potent as gentamicin. Cilantro seeds have actually been used by traditional "food as medicine" practitioners to prevent dysentery for years.

Dr. Kubo explains that many compounds in cilantro show similar activity, and these may act synergistically. There may also be more antibacterial components in other salsa ingredients, which include tomatoes, onions and green chilies. The study suggests that people should eat more salsa with their food, especially fresh salsa.

NEW FOOD CURE?

In reality, it is probably impossible to eat as much cilantro as you would need to offer practical protection against food poisoning. However, Dr. Kubo notes that these new findings may lead to the expanded use of dodecenal as a safe, natural food additive to help prevent food-borne illness. Researchers speculate that the food industry may try to develop and market some form of dodecenal, and it may one day show up as a protective coating for meats or as a disinfectant to be used in cleaning and hand-washing.

In the meantime, some cilantro is better than none. Enjoy your salsa and continue to follow the rules of safe handling, cooking and storage of food.

Supercharge Your Immunity with Just a Few Herbs

James A. Duke, PhD, botany, and adjunct faculty at Tai Sophia Institute, a center for patient care and graduate education in complementary medicine, Laurel, MD. He is a leading authority on medicinal plants and former chief of the US Department of Agriculture Plant Laboratory. He is author of *Dr. Duke's Essential Herbs: 13 Vital Herbs You Need to Disease-Proof Your Body, Boost Your Energy, and Lengthen Your Life*. Rodale.

Medicinal herbs are rich in antioxidants that maintain health and slow the aging process. They also can prevent or alleviate age-related problems, such as arthritis, high blood pressure and failing vision.

We questioned world-renowned botanist James A. Duke, PhD, about which herbs are essential to healthy aging. Dr. Duke has a half-acre medicinal herb garden on his six-acre homestead in Fulton, Maryland.

While these herbs have few significant side effects and are far safer than most synthetic drugs, it is always wise to consult your doctor before treating a medical problem yourself.

Some herbs can interact with prescription and nonprescription drugs, magnifying or weakening their effects. In addition, some people may be allergic to herbs. Be alert to symptoms, such as a rash, when taking any herb.

With your doctor's approval, you can take these herbs all at the same time, along with vitamins, if you wish. Here are eight potent herbs that Dr. Duke uses himself. Follow the dosages suggested on the labels.

BILBERRY: VISION DISORDERS

Bilberry is rich in *anthocyanins*, chemicals that keep the capillary walls strong and flexible. It also is loaded with antioxidants that defend delicate tissue against free-radical damage.

In particular, bilberry protects the retina and its blood supply, preventing and improving vision disorders, such as macular degeneration.

Bilberry can ward off other eye problems, too, including cataracts, glaucoma and poor night vision.

CELERY SEED: GOUT AND ARTHRITIS

I have a special fondness for this herb, which has protected me from agonizing attacks of gout for the last seven years. It lowers blood levels of uric acid as effectively as *allopurinol*, the drug commonly prescribed for gout.

Celery seed, available in capsule form, also contains 25 anti-inflammatory compounds that can reduce the pain and swelling of arthritis. It has chemicals that make blood vessels relax and open, helping to alleviate high blood pressure and angina (chest pain caused by deficient blood flow to the heart).

In folk medicine, celery seed is reputed to be a digestive aid. It is used to relieve gas as well as heartburn, though this has yet to be clinically proven.

ECHINACEA: COLDS AND FLU

This popular herbal medicine is a powerful ally against colds and flu. The purple coneflower from which it comes has been used medicinally by Native Americans for centuries. At least three of the chemicals it contains—*caffeic acid, echinacoside* and *cichoric acid*—have known antiviral properties. In addition, echinacea increases the body's own infection-fighting powers.

Take echinacea at the first sign of an upper-respiratory infection or flu. I also take it when I know I'll be in crowds or around other sources of infection.

This is not an herb for everyday use—the immune system eventually could stop responding to it. I don't take it for more than eight weeks in a row.

GARLIC: BLOOD PRESSURE AND CHOLESTEROL

This pungent bulb was prescribed by Hippocrates, the fifth-century BC Greek physician, and cited as a cure-all in an ancient Sanskrit manuscript. Today, we attribute its medicinal powers to a high concentration of sulfur compounds.

Garlic lowers blood pressure and cholesterol. There also is evidence that it can reduce the risk of cancer, particularly in the gastrointestinal tract.

Garlic contains at least 25 germ-killing compounds and fights bacterial, viral and fungal infections.

Eat at least one raw clove or four cooked cloves daily...or take garlic capsules.

HAWTHORN: POTENT HEART DRUG

An extract made from this flowering shrub can be useful against irregular heart rhythm, angina and shortness of breath. Hawthorn contains seven compounds known to prevent dangerous clotting and three that lower blood pressure. One study at University of Madras in India suggests that hawthorn also may reduce cholesterol.

MILK THISTLE: LIVER PROTECTION

The liver, the organ vital to detoxifying the blood, is under constant assault by pollution. Alcohol, also, is bad for the liver. Milk thistle, a relative of the artichoke, appears to protect the liver. It contains *silymarin,* which strengthens cell membranes and boosts the organ's ability to repair itself. Milk thistle even has been used to treat hepatitis A and C.

I take milk thistle capsules when I'm traveling and will be exposed to smog. If I lived in a major city with pollution problems, I would take it every day.

I also take it before a celebration, when I may be drinking a bit more alcohol than usual.

You can take silymarin capsules or eat milk thistle seeds, available in health-food stores, as you would sunflower seeds.

SAW PALMETTO: PROSTATE PROBLEMS

At least half of men over age 50 have difficulty urinating because benign prostate enlargement chokes off the flow. An extract of saw palmetto, a tropical shrub, has been used for years to treat this problem. A review in the *Journal of the American Medical Association* concluded that saw palmetto facilitates urination in men with prostate problems about as well as medication. Natural chemicals in the herb appear to block a testosterone-type hormone that promotes prostate growth. Men without prostate problems may choose to take it as a preventive measure.

Saw palmetto also may slow down male pattern baldness.

TURMERIC: HEART AND ARTHRITIS

This spice, made from the root of the tropical plant *Curcuma longa,* is a common ingredient in mustard and Indian food—it's what makes curry bright yellow. Turmeric is packed with antioxidants and contains powerful anti-inflammatory compounds called COX-2 inhibitors—the power behind arthritis drugs like Celebrex.

Some research suggests turmeric can stop inflammation about half as effectively as steroids such as cortisone—but without the troubling side effects. This makes it a valuable ally against arthritis. In addition, turmeric protects the heart. It makes blood platelets less likely to clump and form dangerous clots. It also fights cholesterol buildup in the arteries.

Turmeric is available as an herbal preparation. You also can add turmeric to your diet when cooking. I like to use it to make a curried celery soup.

WHICH BRANDS TO BUY

Herbal products are sold by many manufacturers, but there is no federal regulation to ensure quality control.

To be safe, select major brands, such as Nature's Herbs, Nature's Way and Solgar. These are available at most supermarkets, drugstores and health-food stores. Buy preparations that clearly indicate on the labels the exact amounts of active ingredients.

Nature's Virus Killers for Colds and Flu

Mark A. Stengler, ND, naturopathic physician...director, La Jolla Whole Health Clinic, La Jolla, CA...adjunct associate clinical professor, National College of Natural Medicine, Portland, OR...author of *The Natural Physician's Healing Therapies* and coauthor of *Prescription for Natural Cures* (both from Bottom Line Books)...and author of the *Bottom Line/Natural Healing* newsletter.

Do you have to get a cold or the flu this coming season? No! This year can be different. With the right preparation, quick intervention and a lineup of powerful, natural virus fighters, there's a good chance that you can enjoy fall and winter without getting sick. *Here's how...*

RELY ON NATURE'S VIRUS KILLERS

If you start to come down with a cold or the flu, my first recommendation is to change your diet. Eat lightly so that your body can focus on healing. For the first 24 hours, consume filtered water, broths and soups with lots of garlic, onions and spices, such as turmeric and cayenne, which relieve congestion, promote circulation and have a natural anti-inflammatory effect. Herbal teas (especially ginger, cinnamon and peppermint) and steamed vegetables also are good choices. When you're feeling better, move toward a more normal diet.

I have found several supplements to be effective for treating colds and flu. Consider taking these when people around you are sick or when you first feel symptoms. You can use one or any combination until you feel better. These also are safe for children when given in dosages of one-quarter to one-half of what I recommend for adults. The bigger the child, the higher the dose you can use.

• **Lomatium dissectum** is a plant once used by Native Americans to fight Spanish flu. Preliminary research shows that lomatium has the ability to prevent viruses from replicating and to stimulate white blood cell activity.

With colds and flu, I often see improvement within 24 hours. In my experience, the only side effect has been an allergic reaction in the form of a measles-like rash in a small percentage of users. This rash disappears a few days after lomatium is discontinued.

Eclectic Institute makes a potent product called Lomatium-Osha (800-332-4372, *www.eclecticherb.com*), which soothes the respiratory tract. This product is 50% alcohol, so take only the dosage recommended on the label. For children, add one-quarter of the adult dosage to hot water and let it sit for five minutes so that the alcohol evaporates.

Women who are pregnant or nursing should not use lomatium.

• **Elderberry,** as shown by research in Israel, can stimulate the immune system, enhance white blood cell activity and inhibit viral replication.

Flu patients have reported significant improvement within 48 hours of taking elderberry. It also helps with colds.

The elderberry used in research studies is Sambucol Black Elderberry Extract from Nature's Way (to find a retailer, call Total Health Discount Vitamins, 800-283-2833). Adults should take two teaspoons four times daily…children, one teaspoon four times daily.

• **Echinacea.** Contrary to recent media reports, extracts from this plant can be effective for treating colds and flu. Echinacea makes the body's own immune cells more efficient in attacking viruses.

The key is using a product that has been processed to contain a high level of active constituents. Ground-up echinacea root or leaves won't do much. The use of alcohol and water by the manufacturer to extract active components is critical to the product's potency.

Also, be sure to use enough (many people don't). Two potent, well-researched products are Echinamide–Fresh Alcohol-Free Echinacea Extract, Natural Berry Flavor…and Echinamide Anti-V Formula Softgels, both by Natural Factors (to find a retailer, call 800-322-8704 or go to *www.naturalfactors.com*). This echinacea has been shown to reduce the length and severity of the common cold.

If you feel a cold or the flu coming on, take 20 drops of liquid extract or two capsules every two waking hours for 24 hours, then cut back to every three waking hours until the illness has passed.

The same company makes a liquid preparation known as Anti-V Formula, which contains Echinamide, lomatium and other virus fighters. It is the most aggressive product for cold and flu from the Natural Factors line and can be used instead of the other supplements. Take 1.5 milliliters (ml) every two waking hours for the first 48 hours and then every three waking hours until the illness is gone.

• **Homeopathic influenzinum** is an intriguing remedy that I have used with success.

Made from active flu strains, it stimulates the body's own defense system to resist infection. It works along the same lines as an oral vaccine, but since it is homeopathic, none of the flu particles are left in the preparation. It can be used for the prevention or treatment of flu and has no side effects.

Take two 30C-potency pellets twice daily for two weeks at the beginning of flu season (in early November). Take two pellets four times a day when you are exposed to flu sufferers or if you start to have symptoms.

It is available from health-food stores and The Vitamin Shoppe (866-293-3367, *www.vitamin shoppe.com*).

•**Oscillococcinum** is another great homeopathic remedy for flu, which is also available from The Vitamin Shoppe, health-food stores or pharmacies.

It can be taken at the first sign of flu and is the number-one–selling homeopathic flu remedy in the US.

•**N-acetylcysteine (NAC).** This nutrient helps thin the mucus that may accompany a cold or the flu. In addition to making you feel better, NAC helps to prevent sinus and more serious chest infections.

A study at University of Genoa, Italy, showed that NAC, when taken as a supplement, could help prevent as well as treat flu. The nutrient increases levels of the powerful antioxidant *glutathione* in the body, which, in turn, improves immune function. NAC is available at any health-food store and many pharmacies.

If you tend to get the flu every year, take 600 milligrams (mg) twice daily when you are around people who have the flu or if you start feeling sick yourself.

•**Vitamin C** enhances the activity of white blood cells. I have found that taking 3,000 to 5,000 mg daily helps fight viral infections. However, some people get diarrhea from this amount. For immediate treatment of symptoms, start with 5,000 mg in divided doses. If loose stools occur, cut back to 3,000 mg (or even less).

How You Can Help Prevent the Common Cold

Moderate exercise may fight colds. In a new finding, researchers studied 115 women who were sedentary and either overweight or obese. Half performed moderate exercise, such as brisk walking, for 30 to 45 minutes five days a week. The other half attended a once-weekly 45-minute stretching class.

Result: Over 12 months, 48% of the stretchers had at least one cold, compared with only 30% of the exercisers.

Theory: Moderate exercise temporarily increases white blood cell production, which may help guard against infection.

Cornelia Ulrich, PhD, associate member/associate professor, Fred Hutchinson Cancer Research Center, Seattle.

What You Need to Know To Protect Yourself from The Deadly Bird Flu

William Schaffner, MD, professor and chairman of the department of preventive medicine at Vanderbilt University School of Medicine, Nashville. An internationally recognized expert on vaccines, Dr. Schaffner has published more than 60 professional articles on the topic.

If you follow the news, you already know there's a chance that a flu pandemic (a global epidemic) is coming and that it may bring death on a massive scale. Federal, state and local agencies already are working up plans for prevention and treatment.

We can't—individually or as a nation—stop such a disease from reaching the US, but we *can* make ourselves safer by taking some smart precautions.

William Schaffner, MD, chairman of the department of preventive medicine at Vanderbilt University Medical Center and one of the world's top experts on infectious diseases, explains how a pandemic might occur and how to build up our defenses…

UNDERSTANDING THE DANGER

There's no way to predict exactly when the feared pandemic might occur—it could be years away. Based on the recent cases of Avian flu in humans in Asia and in birds in Europe and the Mideast, it might be as soon as next year—it could even be this year. A pandemic can occur at any time of the year, but it is more likely during the traditional flu season and could last a few years.

How the danger started: Eight years ago in Hong Kong, a deadly flu strain that normally affects birds began infecting a few humans as well. According to the World Health Organization, at least 116 people have been infected since 2003, mainly in Thailand and Vietnam. About half of them have died. Avian flu is no longer just Asia's problem—Romania, Turkey and Greece have just confirmed that avian flu has been found among birds there as well.

CHILLING DISCOVERY

Scientists recently discovered that the flu virus that ravaged the world in the 1918 Spanish flu pandemic also was derived from a bird flu virus. That devastating global outbreak killed 50 million people.

Unlike the 1918 virus, the current avian virus is not easily transmitted from person to person. With only a few exceptions, its victims have been infected by coming in direct contact with live infected birds, typically chickens or waterfowl, such as geese or ducks. But influenza viruses have a remarkable ability to mutate. The avian flu virus could change into something much more contagious to humans, then start spreading—within days, thanks to airplane travel. A deadly pandemic then could hit within weeks or months.

WHAT TO DO TODAY

Important steps that you can take to protect yourself against a flu pandemic…

●**Quit smoking.** If you required one more reason, this is it. Smoking irritates the bronchial tubes, making them more vulnerable to any germs that find their way into the throat, including those that can cause avian flu. Smokers also have a harder time fighting any diseases that they do contract.

●**Maintain a healthy weight.** Carrying extra pounds puts unnecessary stress on your heart and lungs, making you more vulnerable to contracting avian flu.

●**Get vaccinated** with a flu shot or the nasal-spray vaccine. The current generation of flu vaccine provides no specific protection against avian flu, but it will help keep your body as strong as possible, improving your odds of survival in case avian flu does strike. Should the pandemic come, those who have been vaccinated but still come down with a flu will know right away that they probably have avian flu. (If you have egg allergies or have had serious reactions to flu shots in the past, talk to your doctor about whether a flu vaccine is safe for you.)

There is a prototype avian flu vaccine that appears to be doing well in clinical trials. Should an avian flu pandemic strike soon, it's possible that this prototype could be rushed into use—but at this point, we don't know how such a vaccine would be distributed…how big a dose would be needed…and how successful it might be against a mutated form of the virus.

●**Take vitamin C.** Some studies suggest that consuming vitamin C supplements and/or foods rich in vitamin C (such as oranges, grapefruits, bell peppers and tomatoes) might help the body avoid viral infections.

●**Stockpile rations for emergencies.** There would probably be a run on supermarkets at the first sign of a pandemic. Maintain a two-week supply of canned foods and water so that you don't have to leave home. This should be enough to last you until a government food-distribution plan is in place, should one be necessary. Other items to have on hand are medications that you take regularly, alcohol wipes and surgical masks.

IF THERE IS AN OUTBREAK…

Should an avian flu pandemic reach the US, stay tuned to TV or radio news for instructions from your health department. There might be quarantines, evacuations or mass vaccination plans in your area.

●**Avoid crowded places.** The best way to remain safe during a pandemic is to limit your exposure to other people. All family members should stay at home as much as possible, avoiding unnecessary trips and visitors. Avoid airplanes, movie theaters and other places where large groups are in close proximity.

It's likely that some employers will tell workers that they can stay home for a time, though other people might have to choose between keeping their jobs and staying home. Local or state governments might close schools.

●**Take precautions** if you must go out during a pandemic. Stay away from anyone who is coughing or sneezing…wash your hands frequently with soap…and carry alcohol wipes to clean your hands after touching anything that has been handled by others.

Many people have asked about wearing cotton surgical masks. There is no evidence that they prevent viral infection, but they are cheap and available at many drugstores. They *might* help, so there's no reason not to wear one.

• **Get to a health-care provider** if the avian flu is in your region and you believe that you're coming down with flulike symptoms—chills, fever, sore throat, fatigue, cough, runny nose, headache or muscle aches. Antiviral drugs are effective only when taken within 48 hours of the onset of your first symptoms.

If possible, obtain your antiviral medication through your doctor's office or a public health office rather than from a hospital. (Your doctor might designate special hours for people with flu symptoms.) During a pandemic, hospitals are likely to be packed with infected people. Your flulike symptoms might mean you just have a cold—but your odds of actually getting avian flu will skyrocket once you enter a hospital handling lots of flu victims.

Are Antibacterial Soaps Making You Sick?

Michael Carlston, MD, former assistant clinical professor of family and community medicine, University of California, San Francisco, School of Medicine.

Consider a mother and a father with four children during the cold and flu season. Inevitably, when one child gets sick, the entire family does. The question is, how do you keep the germ of the day from knocking out the whole household?

According to Michael Carlston, MD, former assistant clinical professor of family and community medicine at the University of California, San Francisco, School of Medicine, the best advice is age-old advice—wash your hands. Wash your hands before eating, before leaving the bathroom and anytime they are dirty, he says. *But, here's the fascinating part of his advice...*

DON'T WASH WITH ANTIBACTERIAL SOAP!

Dr. Carlston's objections to using antibacterials is not that these products don't work, but that they work too well.

Dr. Carlston explains that antibacterials get rid of the "friendly" bacteria that humans need. What remains are the more virulent strains that can harm us, minus a lot of the "friendlies" that protect us from the dangerous ones. The use of antibacterial soap actually puts people at a disadvantage. In a study published recently in the *Annals of Internal Medicine,* researchers found that subjects who used antibacterial soap got just as many runny noses and upper respiratory illnesses as those who did not.

GETTING SICK CAN BE GOOD FOR YOU

Dr. Carlston cautions about becoming overly "germphobic" as the cold and flu season wears on, and wants you to realize that if you do get sick, it is not a totally bad thing. "There is a utility to getting sick," he says. When you get a little illness, such as a cold, it gives your immune system a chance to exercise its illness-fighting ability just as exercising your muscles does. Like muscle, if you don't use it, you lose it. An immune system that never gets the chance to respond to a challenge will not grow stronger.

Of course, he is not recommending that people go out looking for illnesses. It is instinctual and correct to avoid being near very sick people. (And, if you must be near them, don't forget to wash your hands!) It's just that a little sickness can make us stronger overall.

BUILDING YOUR IMMUNITY

Dr. Carlston notes that the average child will get about 10 colds in the first 18 months of life, but then he/she will get far fewer after that. This is because his immune system has learned how to respond. As adults, he says, our immune systems still need the exercise. Of course, this does not apply to those who are immunosuppressed by HIV or other illnesses—they must be extremely careful about avoiding germs.

For the rest of us, though, taking care of ourselves overall (eating nutritious food, exercising regularly, drinking plenty of water and washing our hands) plus catching a cold once in a while may be the best prescription for ongoing health.

Sinus Infection Relief

A new sinus mist reduces repeat sinus infections. SinuNEB uses an inhaler called a nebulizer to convert antibiotics into a fine, inhalable mist that coats the lining of the sinus cavities.

Recent study: Patients with chronic sinusitis remained infection-free an average of 17 weeks after treatment, compared with only six weeks for patients who had undergone surgeries and were treated with antibiotics. SinuNEB also caused fewer side effects, such as upset stomach and diarrhea, than commonly prescribed antibiotics.

Winston C. Vaughan, MD, director and founder, California Sinus Institute, Palo Alto, CA.

How to Eat Fruits and Vegetables Safely

Marion Nestle, PhD, is Paulette Goddard professor of nutrition, food studies and public health at New York University in New York City. She is author or editor of five books, including *What to Eat*. North Point.

I n the wake of a *Salmonella* or *E. coli* outbreak from contaminated fruits or vegetables, many Americans just stop eating the offending fruit or vegetable or become more rigorous in washing it. However, there are probably few people who adopt long-term strategies to protect themselves against dangerous contaminants that could be found in any fruits or vegetables.

WHY OUR FOOD IS AT RISK

Concern about safety should not prevent you from eating fruits and vegetables—as the health benefits of produce far outweigh the risks. Nevertheless, health officials estimate that each year, foodborne bacteria, parasites and viruses sicken 76 million Americans, resulting in 325,000 hospitalizations and 5,000 deaths.

Contaminated fresh produce is the number-one cause of individual cases of foodborne illnesses, according to the Washington, DC–based consumer-advocacy group Center for Science in the Public Interest.

In the US, the safety of fruits and vegetables falls under the jurisdiction of the Food and Drug Administration (FDA). However, in general less than 2% of imported food products is inspected by the FDA, and domestic produce is rarely inspected at all.

The FDA and US Department of Agriculture (USDA) guidelines for the safe handling of produce—known as "Good Agricultural Practices"—suggest methods to help prevent contamination with dangerous microorganisms from water, soil, manure or unhygienic food handlers.

However, these guidelines are voluntary—fruit and vegetable companies do not have to follow them. What's more, the reality is that the FDA does not have the financial resources or personnel to effectively monitor industry practices or the safety of the 741 pounds of produce that are consumed, on average, by every person in the US each year.

Fruits and vegetables are grown in what the FDA typically calls "nonsterile environments"— that is, they grow in dirt. If they come in contact with feces of grazing cattle, wild animals or birds, farm workers or any other source, they can become contaminated with potentially harmful microorganisms. This is obviously unappetizing, and fecal contamination causes health problems if the microorganisms are dangerous types.

BEST SELF-DEFENSE STRATEGIES

Most produce is safe to eat, but regardless of where you shop, there's no way to be 100% certain that the fruits and vegetables you are buying are free of contamination from dangerous microbes.

To do the best you can to protect yourself and your family from unsafe produce, follow these simple steps…

●**Be sure to remove the outer leaves of leafy greens.** That's the area that is most likely to come in contact with manure or other sources of dangerous contamination while leafy vegetables are growing in soil or processed after harvesting.

Caution: The FDA does not require food safety procedures to be followed for most produce, and this includes leafy greens, such as spinach and lettuce, as well as tomatoes and carrots.

Sprouts are an exception. They must be grown under strict safety rules, and problems with them have declined since those precautions went into effect.

• **Store produce in the refrigerator, and wash it before eating.** Harmful microorganisms can multiply on fresh fruits and vegetables, especially when they are transported great distances, sit in supermarket produce bins for extended periods and are not kept cold enough.

Best way to wash produce: Thoroughly rinse produce under running cool tap water. In addition, carefully scrub firm-skinned fruits and vegetables, such as apples and cucumbers, with a clean vegetable brush.

Be sure to clean the vegetable brush, utensils and other kitchen tools in hot water (or the dishwasher) after each use.

Caution: It is a good idea to wash bagged lettuce, spinach and other vegetables—even if the bag says the contents have been "triple washed." If the bags were not kept cold, bacteria could have multiplied inside the package.

To be extra safe, rinse off the inedible rinds of fruits, such as cantaloupe and avocados. If microbes are on the rind, the fruit inside can become contaminated when the rind is pierced by a knife.

Helpful: Do not splurge on expensive fruit and vegetable washes sold in supermarket produce departments. There is no evidence that these special washes are more effective than chlorinated tap water.

Important: Although washing helps protect against foodborne illness from produce, the only way to *guarantee* that fruits and vegetables do not contain harmful microbes is to cook them in boiling water.

• **Buy certified organic.** Studies show that certified organic produce, which is grown in composted manure instead of chemical fertilizers, is no more likely to be contaminated with microbes than conventionally grown produce. That's because, to obtain organic certification, farmers must follow strict rules to ensure that harmful microbes in manure are destroyed (typically through a high-heat decontamination process). Growers of conventional produce are not required to follow such rules.

Organic produce is also a good option if you want to avoid synthetic pesticides and other chemicals that are typically used to kill insects in conventionally grown crops. These chemicals do not reduce your risk for contamination with bacteria and other microbes.

In addition, some research shows that organic produce may be superior to conventionally grown produce in its nutritional value.

Important: When buying organic produce, be sure that it is labeled with a "USDA organic" seal. This means that the producers follow organic growing rules established by the USDA Organic Standards Board and have been inspected by agencies licensed by the USDA to make sure the rules are followed.

Because organic produce is usually more expensive than nonorganic varieties, most people don't buy organic all of the time. The Environmental Working Group (or EWG), a Washington, DC–based, nonprofit environmental research organization, recommends buying organic varieties of produce whose nonorganic counterparts are typically highest in pesticides.

These include peaches, apples, sweet bell peppers, celery, nectarines, strawberries, cherries, pears, imported grapes, spinach, lettuce and potatoes. For a list of other fruits and vegetables evaluated by the EWG, go to the group's Web site, *www.foodnews.org.*

• **Buy from local farmers.** When food is shipped from far away and/or stays in the supermarket for long periods before being sold and eaten, there is more time for microbes to multiply.

Example: If you live on the East Coast, some of the produce in your supermarket sits on a truck for 10 days to two weeks after being harvested in California.

Locally grown foods are fresher and taste better, but there are no guarantees that they are safe. Like any produce, they can come in contact with harmful microbes in the field or during handling, so washing is still essential. And as always, the only way to ensure perfect safety is to cook the foods before eating them.

Important: If you grow your own produce, use a fence to prevent pets and wild animals from defecating in your garden, and be sure to wash everything that you've grown.

If you visit pick-your-own farms for apples, berries, pumpkins or other seasonal produce, be sure to wash these foods, too.

Better Weight Loss

In a study of 147 men and women who ate a reduced-calorie diet for a year, those who consumed 10.5 fluid ounces of low-fat, low-calorie soup twice a day lost 50% more weight than those who ate healthful but carbohydrate-rich snacks, such as baked chips or pretzels.

Theory: Although the soup had the same number of calories as the other snacks, the soup's greater weight and volume made study participants feel full enough to eat less for the rest of the day.

Self-defense: Consume a large mugful of a broth-based, low-fat, low-calorie, low-sodium soup rich in vegetables and/or beans as a first course twice daily.

Barbara Rolls, PhD, professor and Guthrie Chair in Nutrition, Pennsylvania State University, University Park. She is author of *The Volumetrics Eating Plan*. Harper.

The Calcium Diet

Michael Zemel, PhD, professor of nutrition and medicine and director of the Nutrition Institute, University of Tennessee, Knoxville. He is coauthor of *The Calcium Key: The Revolutionary Diet Discovery That Will Help You Lose Weight Faster*. Wiley.

Why are two out of three Americans overweight? Certainly we are eating more and exercising less. But there is another cause—a lack of the mineral calcium in our diets.

If you are among the Americans getting the lowest average level of calcium—255 milligrams (mg) per day—you are 84% more likely to be overweight than if you are among those getting the highest average level—1,346 mg per day—according to an analysis of data from the government's Health and Nutrition Examination Survey.

Simply by getting adequate calcium in our diets, as many as four out of five of us could lose the extra weight.

CALCIUM AND YOUR FAT CELLS

Calcium does far more than just keep your skeleton strong. Without enough calcium circulating in your bloodstream, your heart wouldn't beat, your blood wouldn't clot, your hormones would not regulate your metabolism and your nerves wouldn't transmit signals.

If calcium levels fall—if you eat a low-calcium diet, for example—the body releases more of the hormone *calcitriol*. Calcitriol increases absorption of calcium in the intestines, so you get the most calcium possible from food.

In addition, it increases reabsorption through the kidneys, so that you lose as little calcium as possible through excretion.

Calcitriol also controls how fat cells work. When you get too little calcium and more calcitriol is released, your fat cells make and store more fat, causing weight gain.

MORE PROOF

In a study we conducted at University of Tennessee, overweight people were put on one of three eating plans for six months.

• **Group 1** ate a diet that was 500 calories below maintenance level—the level at which you neither gain nor lose weight—and had no more than one serving of dairy a day for a total of 400 to 500 mg of dietary calcium.

• **Group 2** ate the same calorie-restricted diet but took an 800-mg calcium supplement for a total of 1,200 to 1,300 mg of calcium.

• **Group 3** also ate the calorie-restricted diet but included three servings of low-fat dairy a day, bringing their total calcium intake to 1,200 to 1,300 mg.

Results: Group 1 lost 6% of total weight… Group 2 lost 7.5%…and Group 3—the dairy group—lost 11%. Group 3 also lost more body fat than the other groups, particularly around the waist area. This is an important finding because a slimmer waist is associated with a lower risk of heart disease, stroke, diabetes and cancer.

This means that adding three servings of low-fat dairy to your diet can…

• **Increase the amount of weight you lose by 70%.**

• **Increase the amount of body fat you lose by 64%.**

• **Help you lose 47% more fat from your belly.**

Other studies have replicated these findings as well. In a 10-year study of 3,000 people ages 18 to 30, researchers at Harvard University found that people who ate three servings of dairy a day had a 60% lower risk of being overweight than those who consumed less calcium.

FOOD vs. SUPPLEMENTS

Studies show that calcium from dairy foods is more effective for weight loss than supplements. Why? Food is a complex mixture of known and unknown components. There is a cooperation among the components that can't be reproduced in a nutritional supplement.

Dairy contains calcium and a host of other biologically active components, including the amino acid *leucine*. Recent research reveals that leucine may increase the ability of muscle to use fat.

WHAT TO DO

To lose an average of one pound per week, you need to cut calorie intake and increase calorie burning by about 500 calories per day, or 3,500 calories per week.

To boost the loss to 1.5 to two pounds, you need three or four servings of dairy a day, for a total of 1,200 to 1,600 mg of calcium. The easiest way to get that is with three servings of no-fat (skim) or low-fat milk (8 ounces per serving), yogurt (8 ounces) or cheese (1.5 or 2 ounces, processed).

Strategy: Have milk before a meal. Studies show that getting a liquid form of dairy before eating helps you feel full sooner at that meal and eat less at the next meal.

If you're lactose intolerant, try yogurt with live cultures or cheese (it has very little lactose) or take a lactase supplement when consuming dairy.

To cut 3,500 calories a week: One brisk, hour-long walk burns about 250 calories. If you do that four times a week, you still need to cut 2,500 calories per week, or about 350 calories a day.

Look for just one or two high-calorie items to eliminate from your daily diet.

Examples: A 12-ounce cola has 150 calories …two tablespoons of full-fat salad dressing, 150…a glazed doughnut, 250…a 4-ounce bagel, 300.

Just eliminating these items will help you lose weight, but if you want to lose even more, try boosting your calcium levels.

More from Dr. Michael Zemel…

Weight-Loss Secret

Yogurt helps you lose weight while protecting muscle.

Recent study: Overweight people who ate three servings of yogurt daily for 12 weeks lost 22% more weight, 61% more body fat and 81% more abdominal fat than people who ate a similar number of calories but no dairy products.

The TV Workout

Exercising while watching TV can help keep you healthy. Whenever a commercial comes on, sit up in your chair with abdominal muscles tight and chest high (avoid arching your back). Keeping your feet shoulder-width apart, lean forward slightly and exhale while pushing up through your heels to a standing position. Then inhale as you slowly sit back down—using your leg muscles for control. Repeat this "sofa squat" throughout the entire commercial break.

Linda Buch, American Council on Exercise certified fitness trainer based in Denver, and coauthor of *The Commercial Break Workout: Trim and Tone Two Minutes at a Time*. Prima Lifestyles.

A Stronger Body in Only 30 Minutes a Week

Fredrick Hahn, president and cofounder of the National Council for Exercise Standards, an organization of exercise, medical and scientific professionals. He is owner of Serious Strength Inc., a Slow Burn strength-training studio in New York City, and coauthor of *The Slow Burn Fitness Revolution*. Broadway. *www.seriousstrength.com*.

We know the benefits of strength training. It will restore muscle…increase bone density…improve balance, decreasing the likelihood of falls…and promote weight loss and cardiovascular fitness. But the conventional strength training requires several hours a week and frequently causes injury.

New, better way: Slow Burn, in which the weights are lifted and lowered with incredible slowness—about 10 seconds up and 10 seconds down. The benefits...

• **It's safer.** Slow lifting reduces injury-causing stress on ligaments, tendons and joints. This means that even the elderly can do it safely.

• **It's more effective.** Without the aid of momentum, more muscle fibers are exercised.

• **It's more efficient.** You can get a complete workout in about 30 minutes each week—compared with at least three hours for conventional lifting.

HOW TO DO IT

In a Slow Burn workout, you complete a set of three to six repetitions of each exercise in 60 to 90 seconds. If you perform 10 exercises, you can complete your workout in approximately 10 to 15 minutes. Two workouts a week are all you need.

To obtain the best results, raise and lower weights at the rate of about one inch per second. Allow a total of about 100 seconds for all repetitions of each exercise—push-ups, leg curls, etc. Breathe normally.

Helpful: Use a metronome to maintain the one-inch-per-second rhythm.

Repeat each exercise until your muscles are fatigued and you can't do another repetition in perfect form. If you pass the 90-second point and feel as though you could keep going, the weights are too light. If you cannot complete three repetitions in 90 seconds, the weights are too heavy. Experiment to find the right weight.

The following program stimulates all muscle groups. Do three to six repetitions of each exercise. For exercises that require switching arms or legs, do three to six repetitions with each arm or leg. You will need adjustable hand and ankle weights. Look for sets that adjust from one to 20 pounds.

• **Push-ups.** Kneel on a towel with both your hands flat on the floor in front of you, shoulder-width apart. Keep your back very straight—don't let it sway or arch.

Take three seconds to lower yourself the first inch and at least seven seconds to lower yourself all the way, until your forehead almost touches the floor. Without resting at the bottom, reverse direction. Don't lock your elbows at the top. Just as soon as your arms are almost straight, reverse and go back down. If kneeling push-ups are too easy, do the regular push-ups, with your toes on the floor.

• **Doorknob squats.** Open a door halfway so that you can grip both knobs. Place a stool or 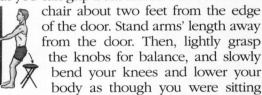 chair about two feet from the edge of the door. Stand arms' length away from the door. Then, lightly grasp the knobs for balance, and slowly bend your knees and lower your body as though you were sitting down. Take three seconds to lower yourself the first inch and seven seconds to go all the way down, until your bottom just touches the stool. Then reverse and rise back up. Be careful not to pull yourself up with your arms—use the muscles of your buttocks and thighs.

• **Side-lying leg lifts.** Try this exercise without ankle weights at first. If it's too easy, start with five-pound weights. Lie on your left side with your head propped on your left hand. Bend your left leg slightly so that your right leg rests on top of the calf. Slowly raise your right leg up toward the ceiling, moving from the hip. Take three seconds to move it the first inch and seven seconds to raise it all the way. Pause at the top, tightly squeeze the hip and buttock muscles for a few seconds, then slowly lower the leg back down. Repeat with the other leg.

• **Single-leg curls.** Attach one five-pound weight to your right ankle. The weight may be too light, but it is a good place to start. Lean forward and put both hands on a stool or chair...keeping your right knee slightly bent and spine straight.

Curl your right leg so that the heel nears your bottom. Take three seconds to curl the leg the first inch and seven seconds to curl it the rest of the way. Pause at the top, squeeze the muscles in the back of your thigh, then slowly reverse direction. Repeat with the other leg.

• **Side shoulder raise and overhead press.** This movement combines two exercises. Start with five-pound dumbbells. With a dumbbell in each hand, sit on a chair with your back straight and your feet flat on the floor. Slowly raise the weights away from both of your sides, taking three seconds to move them the first inch and seven seconds to raise them until they're parallel to the floor. Pause at the top for a few seconds, then slowly lower the weights.

Without resting, move to the second phase of the exercise. Elbows bent, hold the weights at shoulder height, then slowly raise them overhead, taking three seconds to move them the first inch and seven seconds to go all the way up. Pause for a second, then gradually lower the weights until they're back at shoulder height. Do not lock your elbows at the top. Let your muscles support the weights.

• **Single-arm back pull-ups.** You need a stool or chair and a six- to eight-pound dumbbell. Hold the dumbbell in your right hand…then face the stool with your left leg forward…and support yourself with your left hand on the stool. Let your right arm hang beside the stool.

Slowly pull the dumbbell back and upward, taking three seconds to move it the first inch and seven seconds to raise it all the way. Your right elbow will be facing up and behind you. Pause at the top, squeeze the arm and back muscles for a few seconds, then lower the weight back down. Don't let your arm hang down at the end of the movement. Keep tension on the muscles all the time. Repeat with the other arm.

• **Biceps curls.** Sit on a stool or straight-back chair with a five-pound dumbbell in each hand. Tuck your elbows into your sides, and keep them there throughout the exercise. The only thing that should move is your lower arm.

Curl the dumbbells up toward your shoulders, taking about three seconds to move them the first inch and seven seconds to curl them all the way. Squeeze the muscles in the forearms and upper arms for a

few seconds at the top of the movement, and then slowly lower the weights back down.

• **Shoulder shrugs.** Sit on a stool or straight-back chair with a 10-pound dumbbell in each hand. Let your arms hang down away from your hips, with the elbows slightly bent.

Then, raise up the tops of your shoulders as though you're trying to touch them to your earlobes. Sit up straight. Don't slouch forward or backward. Take three seconds to move your shoulders the first inch and seven seconds to raise them as far as they'll go. Pause at the top to squeeze the muscles in your shoulders, then lower them back down.

• **Abdominal crunches.** Lie on your back with your feet flat on the floor and your knees bent at a 90° angle. Tuck a rolled towel under your lower back…hold your arms straight in front of you…and keep your chin tucked into your chest. Curl your torso upward and forward, taking three seconds to move the first inch and seven seconds to move forward. Do not try to sit all the way up. Keep your lower back in contact with the towel. Pause and squeeze abdominal muscles at the top of the movement, then slowly lower your torso down. Don't rest your shoulders on the floor at the end. As soon as they brush the floor, repeat the exercise.

Illustrations by Shawn Banner.

Exercises That Help With Everything You Do

Larkin Barnett, adjunct professor of exercise science at Florida Atlantic University in Boca Raton, and author of *Functional Fitness: The Ultimate Fitness Program for Life on the Run.* Florida Academic.

Functional training is a form of exercise that strengthens the muscles that we use in everyday activities, such as standing, walking, sitting, doing chores and carrying packages.

How it works: Functional training helps integrate the limbs and the trunk muscles for fluid, powerful movements…puts your body into proper alignment…improves posture and balance …and promotes deep breathing for relaxation.

A functional fitness routine can be incorporated into cardiovascular and strength-training workouts. *The exercises described below are designed for people of all fitness levels and should be performed daily…*

SIT UP AND TAKE NOTICE

Benefits: Corrects trunk alignment, including weak abdominal muscles that don't provide sufficient support for the lower back…and enhances stamina and endurance.

Good for: Carrying objects…walking and running…and relieving muscle tension caused by working at a desk or a computer.

What to do: While sitting in a straight-backed chair, scrunch your shoulders up toward your ears, then relax them. Inhale slowly while you raise your shoulders, then exhale slowly as you lower them. Do this three to five times, feeling tension drain out of your shoulders and neck.

Next, sit tall, perched on your sit-bones (you can locate these by rocking side-to-side) and concentrate on stacking your hips, ribs, chest and head on top of each other like building blocks. Exhale powerfully while pulling your abdominal muscles inward toward your spine. Then pull your shoulders back gently. Take several deep breaths.

Finally, sit up tall, while picturing the tops of your ears stretching upward. This elongates the spine and improves respiratory function. Tighten your abdominals inward and upward toward your spine while exhaling forcefully three to five times.

THE COMPASS

Benefits: Strengthens your postural muscles (to improve coordination and balance)…and reduces fatigue and stress on the legs, hips and back.

Good for: Relieving muscle soreness from extended standing as well as improving performance in all sports and physical activities.

What to do: With your feet flat on the ground about 12 inches apart, pretend you're standing in the middle of a large compass. With exaggerated movements, shift your entire body toward each of the four main points on the compass—north (forward), south (backward), east (to the right) and west (to the left)—pausing momentarily at each point. Do this three to five times. Contract your abdominal muscles and notice how your control improves.

Gradually make your movements smaller and smaller. Do this for 30 seconds. End by standing still and feeling your body weight evenly distributed.

THE PELVIS AS A FISH BOWL

Benefits: Centers the hips and places the pelvis in neutral alignment, reducing stress on the legs, back and neck.

Good for: Lifting…getting in and out of bed… and swinging a golf club or tennis racket.

What to do: Standing with your feet about 12 inches apart, contract your stomach muscles and draw them inward and up toward your spine. Picture your hips as a fish bowl filled with water, with the bowl's rim at your waistline.

Now tip your hips forward slightly and visualize water spilling out of the front of the fish bowl. Next, tip your hips backward slightly and visualize water sloshing out of the back of the bowl. Finally, balance the fish bowl so that the rim is perfectly level. This is your pelvis's "neutral" position. Throughout the day, assume this position as you stand up, walk and sit.

SHOULDER BLADE, ARM, FINGERTIP

Benefits: Teaches you to initiate arm movements from your trunk muscles (including your shoulder girdle muscles) for more power and control.

Good for: Relieving muscle tension caused by driving a car or speaking on the telephone…and playing golf and racket sports.

What to do: While standing, lift your arms to your sides at shoulder level. Then lift your arms higher, in the shape of a "U," while sliding your shoulder blades downward. Imagine that you have a balloon next to each ear. Initiate these movements from the shoulder blades. Lower your arms, then repeat three to five times.

Illustrations by Shawn Banner.

Vinegar May Help Fight Diabetes

In a recent study, healthy patients and patients with a prediabetic condition known as insulin resistance drank a vinegar drink (⅛ cup of vinegar, diluted with ¼ cup of water and sweetened with saccharine) or a placebo drink before a high-carbohydrate meal.

The vinegar treatment improved insulin sensitivity by up to 40% in both groups.

Theory: Vinegar inhibits the breakdown of carbohydrates, thereby decreasing the blood glucose spikes that occur in people with diabetes.

If you are diabetic or insulin resistant: Talk to your doctor about drinking diluted vinegar before meals.

Carol S. Johnston, PhD, RD, professor and nutrition department chair, Arizona State University East, Mesa.

Reduce Diabetic Nerve Pain

Mark A. Stengler, ND, naturopathic physician…director, La Jolla Whole Health Clinic, La Jolla, CA…adjunct associate clinical professor, National College of Natural Medicine, Portland, OR…author of *The Natural Physician's Healing Therapies* and coauthor of *Prescription for Natural Cures* (both from Bottom Line Books)…and author of the *Bottom Line/Natural Healing* newsletter.

Researchers evaluated the effects of the nutritional supplement acetyl-L-carnitine (ALC) on diabetic neuropathy, a condition that occurs when diabetes damages the nerves, especially those in the hands, legs and feet. Symptoms include numbness, tingling and/or pain.

New study: In two clinical trials, 1,257 people with diabetes took 1,500 milligrams (mg) of ALC, 3,000 mg of ALC or a placebo pill daily for one year.

Those who took 3,000 mg of ALC daily experienced a significant reduction in pain.

My view: While ALC often is prescribed for those with age-related cognitive decline (poor memory) and early-stage Alzheimer's disease, it

now should be considered a primary form of treatment for diabetic neuropathy.

Take 1,000 mg of ALC three times daily (the same dosing schedule used in the study).

ALC has a blood-thinning effect, so check with your doctor before using it if you take a blood thinner, such as *warfarin* (Coumadin).

Protect Yourself from Killer Bacteria

Edward K. Chapnick, MD, director of the division of infectious diseases at Maimonides Medical Center in Brooklyn, NY, and associate professor of medicine at Mount Sinai School of Medicine in New York City. He has published more than 30 medical journal articles on infectious diseases.

Imagine entering a hospital for heart surgery, a joint replacement or some other procedure. The treatment is successful, but you contract an infection during your hospital stay.

Each year, this happens to two million Americans. The infection is usually minor—a simple rash and fever that can be cured with antibiotics. But about 10% of hospital-acquired infections are serious. Some bacteria are resistant to most—if not all—antibiotics, and harmful organisms can quickly invade the bloodstream and harm the skin, organs, muscles and/or bones. More than 90,000 Americans die of these hospital-acquired infections annually.

While most hospitals have stepped up their efforts to prevent infections, only recently have many patients become aware that they must be more assertive in protecting themselves.

HOW TO AVOID BACTERIA

Bacteria can live for hours—sometimes even days—on almost any surface and then transfer easily to skin. From there, bacteria can enter the body through breaks in the skin or via touching the eyes, nose or mouth. Hand-washing is the most effective way to help prevent the spread of bacteria and other infection-causing organisms. (For more on hand-washing, see the following article.)

Other ways to protect yourself—or a loved one…

●**Ask doctors and nurses to disinfect medical devices.** To prevent the spread of bacteria or other germs, stethoscopes, blood pressure cuffs and other such medical devices should be cleaned with a disinfectant alcohol wipe before they touch your skin.

●**Avoid touching surfaces touched by other people.** Some people do their best to avoid touching tabletops, chairs, elevator doors or any other surface. If this is impractical, use alcohol-based disinfectant gels and/or wipes. To prevent a possible infection, avoid rubbing bare skin from any part of your body against these surfaces. In a recent study, about three-quarters of hospital rooms tested were contaminated with bacteria.

●**Be aware that visitors can carry germs into your hospital room.** Ask visitors not to sit on your bed—they can transfer bacteria from their clothes to the sheets…or use the bathroom in your room—they can transfer germs to bathroom surfaces. Even doctors' neckties can carry bacteria or other germs, research shows.

Hospital patients typically are at greater risk of contracting an infectious disease due to their weakened immunity, but it's also wise for hospital visitors to follow hygienic practices to avoid getting sick.

PREP YOURSELF

Patients themselves often carry bacteria, such as *Staphylococcus aureus* (staph), on their bodies and/or clothes when they check into the hospital. These germs don't always cause symptoms—up to 30% of healthy adults carry staph on their skin. However, if your skin is colonized with bacteria when you go for surgery, it can enter your body at the surgical site. *To protect yourself…*

●**Wash your body.** Three to five days before surgery, start showering or bathing daily using a special 4% chlorhexidine soap. Chlorhexidine is a powerful antiseptic agent that will help remove bacteria from the skin's surface. Chlorhexidine soap (such as Hibiclens or Betasept) is available over the counter at most drugstores. If it is not in stock, ask the pharmacist to order it.

Caution: Because this soap can irritate the skin or cause an allergic reaction in some people, do not use the soap for more than five days…avoid the use of other skin products during that time…

and be sure that your doctor gives his/her consent to use the soap.

●**Do not shave.** No matter how careful you are, shaving causes microscopic nicks in your skin. Any break in the skin can potentially create an entry point for bacteria. For 72 hours before surgery, do not shave the surgical site, even if the site is on your legs, underarms or face. If your surgery typically requires shaving, ask your doctor if clippers can be used instead of a razor by hospital personnel before your surgery.

●**Ask for a staph test.** A week to 10 days before surgery, ask your surgeon to test you for *methicillin-resistant Staphylococcus aureus* (MRSA) by getting a nasal swab. If the swab shows that you are a carrier of the bacterium, specific infection-control procedures are used in the hospital. A topical antibiotic might also be prescribed.

Helpful: Almost everyone will be given an oral antibiotic within 60 minutes of receiving surgery to help prevent an infection. However, it's common for busy hospital staff to forget this routine medication. Be sure to remind your doctor.

If you're scheduled for surgery: Call your state's health department and ask if hospitals in the state are required to report infection rates. If so, get the latest report for the hospital where you'll be treated. Discuss any findings with your doctor.

CATHETERS AND IVs

Having a catheter or intravenous (IV) line increases your risk for infection because bacteria from your own body or a health-care worker's hands can enter at the insertion site. Catheters are tubes that are used to drain liquids, such as urine, from the body. IV lines deliver fluids, such as medication and nutrients, directly into a vein. *You may not have a choice whether or not a catheter or IV is inserted, but always ask…*

●**Why is the catheter and/or IV there?** Often, a catheter or IV is used when a patient enters the emergency room, but is then forgotten for a time after it is no longer needed. If you don't know why you have a catheter or IV, ask.

●**How many days will I need the catheter and/or IV?** The answer largely depends on your condition, but it's important to let your doctor know that you want a catheter and/or IV removed as soon as possible. With urinary catheters, the risk for an infection increases by at least 5% each day it remains in place. That means that it should come out as soon as medically possible.

Helpful: Every day, ask your nurse or doctor whether the catheter can come out...don't wait for medical staff to think of removing it.

With peripheral IVs (the kind that are inserted into a vein in your hand or arm), the risk for infection is relatively low until the third or fourth day. If an IV has been in place for four days, ask when you are scheduled to have it replaced with a new one. (Central venous lines, which are inserted in large veins of the neck or chest, don't have the same risk and can stay in place almost indefinitely.)

More from Dr. Edward Chapnick...

Hand-Washing Secrets

If you are hospitalized, everyone who enters your room should wash his/her hands. This includes family members, doctors, nurses and other hospital staff. If you feel embarrassed to remind your doctor or anyone else, raise the issue as a question: "Did you remember to wash your hands?"

Be sure that people who wash with soap and water dry their hands with a clean paper towel and not a cloth towel from the bathroom in your hospital room. The paper towel should also be used to turn off the faucet.

In most hospitals, alcohol-based hand-cleaning gel dispensers are mounted on the wall in or near each patient's room—these are for everyone to use, not just staff. These gels (which should contain at least 62% alcohol) are superior to hand-washing at killing germs. Alcohol dries out the skin less than soap and water does, so it is best for frequent cleanings. If hands are visibly soiled, soap and water must be used.

Important: Latex gloves are meant to protect the person wearing them, not the patient. If hands aren't washed before putting on gloves, bacteria will live on the gloves. If a hospital staff member enters your room already wearing gloves, ask him to remove the gloves, clean his hands and put on a fresh pair.

How Safe Are Your Vitamins and Minerals?

Tod Cooperman, MD, president and founder of ConsumerLab.com, White Plains, NY, which provides the latest testing results and issues warnings and information about recalls approximately every two weeks. He is the editor of *Health, Harm or Rip-Off?* Bottom Line Books.

The FDA requires nutritional supplement labels to state exactly what's contained in the package. But government inspectors rarely check.

Result: Many supplements contain too little or too much of the active ingredient...are contaminated with pesticides or heavy metals (arsenic, cadmium, lead)...or aren't properly absorbed by the body.

ConsumerLab.com, an independent evaluator of nutritional and vitamin/mineral supplements, recently tested more than 500 products in laboratories throughout the country to determine if their ingredients matched what was listed on the label. Products also were tested for contamination and their ability to dissolve in the body.

Best choices...*

MULTIVITAMINS/MINERALS

Most people use multivitamins and minerals as "nutritional insurance" to compensate for gaps in their diets.

Test results: Of the 27 products tested, nine failed. The most common problems were related to vitamin A. Some of the products contained more than 150% of the amount listed on the label.

Excessive vitamin A can cause headache, anemia and bone and liver damage. Other multivitamin formulas contained lower-than-listed levels of beta-carotene and folic acid, an essential nutrient for preventing birth defects.

Reliable products include...

• **Geritol Complete.**

• **Life Essentials Dietary Supplement.**

• **Nutrilite Daily Multivitamin and Multimineral Dietary Supplement.**

*Other approved products may display a seal of approval from ConsumerLab.com, the US Pharmacopeia (USP) or NSF International. All these organizations evaluate supplements. Be sure to check with your doctor for the dosages that are right for you.

- **Ocuvite Zinc with Key Antioxidants Vitamin and Mineral Supplement.**

B VITAMINS

The eight B vitamins are involved in all aspects of metabolism, but your body can't produce them. B vitamins are available only through food or supplements. Some supplements contain a single B vitamin, while others contain all eight.

Test results: Of the 21 products tested, nine listed doses on their labels that were in excess of the safe upper limit (UL) for vitamin B-3 (niacin), as established by the Institute of Medicine of the National Academies.

High doses can be taken under a doctor's supervision to safely lower cholesterol. But people who take a B-complex supplement that contains 35 milligrams (mg) of niacin or more may experience side effects, such as facial flushing and skin tingling. At very high doses, niacin can cause liver damage.

Reliable products include…

- **Nature Made Balanced B-150 B-Complex Supplement Time Released**
- **Nutrilite Natural B Complex Dietary Supplement**
- **Stresstabs High Potency B-Complex with Antioxidants C & E & Folic Acid + Zinc Dietary Supplement**
- **Vitamin World B-100 Ultra B-Complex, 100 mg**

VITAMIN C

It's an antioxidant that may boost immune function, reduce cataracts and other eye diseases and protect against cancer.

Test results: Of the 26 products tested, one failed to dissolve properly and three didn't contain enough vitamin C.

Reliable products include…

- **Kirkland Signature Vitamin C with Rose Hips, 1,000 mg**
- **Nature Made Vitamin C, 1,000 mg**
- **Nature's Bounty Natural Vitamin C, 1,000 mg**
- **Nutrilite Bio C Plus, 250 mg**

Helpful: Don't spend extra money for natural forms of vitamin C. Synthetic and natural forms have the same effects in the body.

VITAMIN E

The amount needed for daily nutrition is easily obtained from foods (nuts, grains, oils, etc.). Higher doses are thought to be beneficial in preventing and/or treating prostate and other cancers, as well as Alzheimer's disease.

Test results: Of the 28 products tested, two had less vitamin E than listed on the label, and one product labeled as "natural" contained synthetic vitamin E.

Important: Natural vitamin E, listed on labels as d-alpha-tocopherol, works more efficiently in the body than the synthetic dl form.

Reliable products include…

- **Brite-Life Natural Vitamin E, 400 international units (IU)**
- **Carlson E-Gems Vitamin E, 400 IU**
- **Solgar Natural Vitamin E, 400 IU**
- **Twinlab E-400 Caps, 100% Natural, 400 IU**

CALCIUM

Most people take this mineral to strengthen their bones, but studies have suggested that it also may reduce the risk for colon polyps.

Test results: Of the 35 products tested, four contained less calcium than the amount that was listed on the label.

Reliable products include…

- **Citracal Ultradense Calcium Citrate, 200 mg**
- **GNC Calcimate Plus 800, 200 mg**
- **Nature's Bounty Calcium Citrate, 200 mg**
- **Puritan's Pride Calcium Citrate, 200 mg**

More from Dr. Tod Cooperman…

Do Your Supplements Really Work?

Vitamin and mineral tablets sometimes fail to dissolve in the body, usually because of poor manufacturing practices. *If you want to test the tablets yourself…*

- **Heat one cup of vinegar** (any type can be used) to about 100°F, keeping the liquid warm and at a steady temperature.

• **Place one vitamin or mineral pill in the cup.** For 30 to 45 minutes, stir the liquid periodically. Try to avoid hitting the pill.

• **If the pill doesn't dissolve within 45 minutes,** it may not dissolve completely when it is in the intestine, which diminishes its effectiveness.

Note: This test does not work for timed-release products and is not necessary to perform on chewables.

Emergency Room Self-Defense

Ted Christopher, MD, chairman, department of emergency medicine at Thomas Jefferson University Hospital, Philadelphia.

Hospital emergency departments (EDs) are busier now than ever. Because of decreasing health-care budgets, examining rooms and equipment are in short supply. Doctors, nurses and technicians are overworked. No wonder the average wait to see a doctor is 49 minutes—with many patients in the ED waiting for hours.

For better emergency care…

• **Call 911 or an ambulance if you suspect heart attack or stroke,** two "time-dependent" conditions that can quickly worsen. Ambulance technicians will begin your care on the way… and you're more likely to be seen by a doctor as soon as you arrive at the hospital.

If your condition isn't truly an emergency, arriving by ambulance won't make a difference, and you could get stuck with paying the bill. The sickest patients always get taken care of first.

• **Go to the closest hospital if you think you have an emergency.** The majority of all hospital EDs are now being staffed with board-certified emergency physicians. Most of the teaching hospitals are staffed with attending emergency physicians and many residents and interns. In nonteaching hospitals, there will be only one or two doctors on staff. You may spend time waiting in either setting.

• **Don't wait for a referral from your doctor.** It is no longer necessary to bring a referral or get prior approval from your doctor before going to the ED.

Everyone who comes to the ED undergoes *triage,* a process by which each patient is evaluated by a nurse to determine how serious his condition is and who is to be seen first by a doctor.

• **Know the names and phone numbers of all your doctors**—especially your primary-care physician, but also any specialists you may have seen. Your private doctors often possess medical information that can assist the emergency physician in treating you.

• **Bring all of your medications.** ED staff will learn a lot about your health history simply by reading the labels. If you're going to need drugs, it's vital that the doctors know what medications you're taking.

Helpful: Keep a list of all your medications, along with the details of other health information (serious allergies, for example), on the refrigerator door. If you're unable to talk, the ambulance crew can take the list to the ED.

Even better: Bring the actual bottles—the printed labels are easiest to read.

• **Report changes in symptoms immediately.** Don't suffer in silence in the waiting room. You'll see a doctor more quickly if you inform the staff that your symptoms are getting worse. You should be given medication, if necessary, even before you see a doctor.

Important Medical Tests Doctors Don't Tell You About

Leo Galland, MD, director, Foundation for Integrated Medicine, which promotes a comprehensive approach to health care, New York City, *www.mdheal.org.* He is author of *The Fat Resistance Diet* (Broadway) and a recipient of the Linus Pauling Award.

The special screening tests—for discovering heart disease, aneurysms, lung cancer and ovarian cancer—could save your life. But there is a good chance that your physician won't order them because insurance companies rarely pay for them.

Reason: Insurance companies typically pay for tests only when you have been diagnosed with a particular condition or when there is a high likelihood that you might have it. With some exceptions, such as mammograms, insurance rarely pays for screening tests aimed at early detection.

Ask your doctor if you should have any of the following tests, even if you have to pay for them yourself. They are available at most diagnostic and medical centers around the country. Ask your doctor for a referral.

These tests are not appropriate for everyone, but early research suggests that they could be lifesavers for those with key risk factors…

CHOLESTEROL TEST

The traditional cholesterol tests only measure HDL ("good") cholesterol and triglycerides. The formula used to calculate levels of harmful LDL cholesterol isn't always accurate. This partly explains why half of people who have heart attacks have cholesterol levels that appear normal.

Better: Expanded cholesterol tests measure LDL specifically, giving more accurate readings. About 40 million American adults have hidden heart disease. Expanded cholesterol tests could identify 95% of these patients before a heart attack occurs.

The tests also look at individual HDL and LDL particles and determine how helpful—or harmful—they are likely to be.

Example: HDL protects against heart disease, so high levels are desirable. But some people who appear to have high levels actually have a subtype of HDL that isn't very helpful. Also, though all LDL particles are bad, the smaller ones are more dangerous than the bigger ones. These kinds of differences just aren't detectable with the conventional tests—but they can be detected with the expanded tests.

Who should consider them: Patients with mildly elevated levels of cholesterol—200 to 230 milligrams per deciliter (mg/dL)—who smoke or who have the cardiovascular risk factors, such as heart problems, high blood pressure or a family history of heart disease.

Cost: $75 to $175.

ANEURYSM TEST

Aneurysms are bulges in artery walls. They can be deadly when they rupture, killing 80% to 90% of people who have ruptured aneurysms. About 30,000 Americans die from this annually.

Better: An aneurysm scan uses an ultrasound wand to detect aneurysms in the abdominal aortic arteries. It's the only noninvasive test that allows doctors to identify aneurysms before they rupture. Surgery to repair aneurysms can increase survival rates to 99%.

Who should consider it: Anyone over age 60 who has cardiovascular risk factors, such as high blood pressure, or who smokes…as well as anyone over age 50 who has a family history of heart disease.

Cost: $60 to $200, depending on the extent of the scan.

HEART DISEASE TEST

Current methods for detecting heart disease risk, such as checking blood pressure, miss up to 75% of patients who later on develop heart problems.

Better: The electron beam tomography, or EBT, heart scan is the first direct, noninvasive way of identifying atherosclerosis, the primary risk factor for heart disease. The patient lies in a dough-nut-shaped machine while the electron beams map out calcium deposits in the arteries. The buildup of calcium indicates the presence of plaque—fatty deposits that hamper blood flow to the heart and increase risk of blood clots. The patients who are found to have early signs of heart disease can take the appropriate steps—such as lowering cholesterol, controlling blood pressure, stopping smoking, etc.—to prevent problems from progressing.

Drawback: Calcium deposits do not always indicate an elevated risk of heart attack. The deposits may be harmless. On the other hand, a person who has a clear scan could actually have dangerous levels of plaque.

Patients with high calcium levels also may have to take a follow-up stress test. If this test is positive, the patient may have to undergo an angiogram—an invasive procedure. If the angiogram shows no heart disease, the patient has undergone these extra tests unnecessarily. Still the EBT is considered useful because traditional tests don't catch most heart problems.

Who should consider it: All men over age 45 and women over age 55. If you have heart disease risk factors—smoking, a family history of heart disease, etc.—consider having an EBT 10 years sooner.

Cost: About $400.

LUNG CANCER TEST

Lung cancer rarely causes symptoms until it reaches an advanced stage. The five-year survival rate is about 15%. Conventional X-rays may fail to detect early-stage tumors.

Better: The spiral CT scan can detect cancerous tumors as small as one grain of rice. Eighty percent of lung cancers spotted in scanning studies were caught at a potentially treatable stage.

Drawbacks: The test can result in false-positives—findings that indicate cancer when none is present. This could lead to unnecessary and risky lung biopsies. The rate of false-positives improves when patients have follow-up scans.

Who should consider it: Smokers as well as former smokers age 50 and over who have smoked at least one pack daily for 10 years or two packs daily for five years.

Cost: $300 to $500.

OVARIAN CANCER

More than 14,000 American women die from ovarian cancer every year. It is one of the deadliest of female cancers. Like lung cancer, it often has no symptoms until it reaches an advanced stage of development.

Better: An ultrasound device inserted into the vagina allows doctors to inspect the ovaries for any malignant changes. University of Kentucky researchers used this test on 23,000 women. Twenty-nine showed cancerous ovarian tumors, 76% of which were detected at an early, more treatable stage. Typically, only 25% of ovarian cancers are caught early.

Drawback: The test isn't able to differentiate between malignant and benign growths—so positive test results could result in unnecessary procedures.

Who should consider it: Women age 45 and older with risk factors, such as a family history of ovarian, breast or colon cancer...or a history of fertility or hormone-replacement treatment...or who never have been pregnant.

Cost: About $250.

Nobel Prize Winner Who Discovered Real Cause of Ulcers Tells All

Barry J. Marshall, MD, senior principal research fellow, School of Biomedical, Biomolecular and Chemical Sciences, University of Western Australia, Perth. He is the winner, with J. Robin Warren, MD, of the 2005 Nobel Prize in Physiology or Medicine and the editor of *Helicobacter Pioneers*. Blackwell Scientific.

When two Australian physician-researchers first suggested that ulcers might be caused by a stomach bug, the medical establishment scoffed.

For decades, doctors had believed that emotional stress prompted the stomach to churn out acid to the point that it literally ate a hole in the stomach lining. Doctors treated the resulting ulcers with antacids—and even psychotherapy to help sufferers relax.

Gastroenterologist Barry J. Marshall, MD, and pathologist J. Robin Warren, MD, speculated that a bacterium, later named *Helicobacter pylori,* or *H. pylori,* was the real culprit.

In 1984, they published their H. pylori report in the British medical journal *The Lancet*. The two doctors won the 2005 Nobel Prize in Physiology or Medicine for their discovery.

To learn more about ulcers, we interviewed Dr. Marshall shortly after he won the Nobel Prize...

●**What made you persist in an area of research that contradicted conventional medical treatments?** After Dr. Warren completed research showing that about half of the patients who underwent stomach biopsies had bacteria that created inflammation in the stomach lining, it was natural for us to continue investigating the role that the bacteria was playing.

Once the connection with ulcers was made, we saw that antibiotics cured 92% of patients no matter how severe their disease. In fact, we found such a high cure rate versus no "cures" in the standard treatment group that we only needed to treat a small number of patients from the standard group to convince ourselves that we were correct.

●**How do you think your winning the Nobel Prize for research on H. pylori will affect ulcer treatment?** Very conservative doctors who do not ordinarily look for H. pylori now may be forced to do so, because their patients may have read about our research in news reports on the Nobel Prize.

•**Why do some individuals with H. pylori develop ulcers and others don't?** You catch H. pylori from family members or contaminated water in developing countries.

For an ulcer to develop, the patient must be able to produce high amounts of stomach acid. When H. pylori is present, the infection-fighting white blood cells attack the bacteria. In doing this, the cells damage the stomach lining, causing inflammation (gastritis) and, years later, an ulcer. Because H. pylori bacteria produce varying levels of toxins, some do not damage the stomach wall enough to cause an ulcer.

•**Aren't some ulcers caused by the use of stomach-irritating painkillers?** Yes. Aside from H. pylori, many aspirin-type drugs, called nonsteroidal anti-inflammatory drugs (NSAIDs), usually taken for arthritis, can lead to ulcers. Approximately 40% of ulcers result from NSAID use. The remainder are due to H. pylori.

•**Does H. pylori ever cause anything more serious than an ulcer?** Yes. The inflammation produced by H. pylori also can lead to stomach cancer.

•**Who should be tested for H. pylori?** Anyone with stomach symptoms, such as pain or burning in the upper stomach, nausea or vomiting. Also, if you have a family history of stomach cancer—in a parent or sibling—you should be tested. The test itself involves drawing a blood sample to test for antibodies or a breath test.

•**If a person tests positive for H. pylori, what's the best treatment?** The best treatment is acid reduction—with proton-pump inhibitors, such as *esomeprazole* (Nexium), *pantoprazole* (Protonix) or *rabeprazole* (AcipHex)—combined with an effective antibiotic. In general, taking an antibiotic, such as *clarithromycin* (Biaxin) with *amoxicillin* (Amoxil), for 10 to 14 days will work.

•**Does eliminating the bacterium pose any risks?** No. However, paradoxically, H. pylori does lower stomach acid levels in some people. In these people, H. pylori protects them somewhat against acid-stimulated diseases in the esophagus, such as gastroesophageal reflux disease (GERD), and, as a result, esophageal cancer. That's because stomach acid leaking up into the esophagus increases cancer risk in that location. However, this should not stop us from treating H. pylori, because both the bacteria and GERD are easily treatable.

•**Some studies have shown that cranberry juice may help fight ulcers. Is this an important discovery?** It is likely that many food products do inhibit H. pylori and, as a result, help ulcers heal. In most cases, however, the effect is not very strong.

•**What areas of research do you think hold the most promise for a cure or new treatment for disease?** Many aspects of H. pylori colonization still are not understood. For example, at least 30% of H. pylori genes have no known purpose. Deciphering these genes will provide important insights into the functioning of the gastrointestinal system. My lab at the University of Western Australia is performing molecular studies to discover new useful genes in our H. pylori strains.

•**Did you or Dr. Warren have any idea that you might win the Nobel Prize?** We knew immediately that we had made an important discovery. In such an underpopulated area as Western Australia, however, we could not imagine how many millions of people would benefit. We dreamed of winning the Nobel Prize but always thought that other recipients over the years were worthy laureates.

You May Have This Stomach Bug and Not Even Know It

Martin J. Blaser, MD, the Frederick H. King professor of internal medicine and chairman and professor of microbiology in the departments of medicine and microbiology at New York University School of Medicine, New York City. He is past president of the Infectious Diseases Society of America and a member of the editorial boards of various medical journals.

Twenty years ago, in a report published in the prestigious British medical journal *The Lancet,* scientists from Australia announced that they had isolated a microorganism that lives on the thick mucous lining of the stomach. They theorized that the bacterium might play a role in chronic active gastritis, a persistent inflammation of the stomach.

Over the next two decades, research into the bacterium—named *Helicobacter pylori,* or *H. pylori*—led to a new era in gastrointestinal medicine. The bacterium was found in the stomachs of more than half the world's population—70% to 90% in developing countries, and about 30% in the US. H. pylori also was discovered to be a leading cause of ulcers and stomach cancer.

These days, a doctor who finds a patient infected with H. pylori attempts to eradicate it. But is that treatment always helpful? Or, as newer studies suggest, is the eradication of H. pylori creating an unexpected and unprecedented epidemic of diseases of the esophagus, the tube that connects the back of the throat to the stomach?

To answer all these and other questions, we spoke to Martin J. Blaser, MD, a renowned authority on H. pylori.

●**Billions of people worldwide are infected with H. pylori. Is this a normal condition or a disease?** The most recent evidence strongly suggests that H. pylori was once even more common than it is now, perhaps found in everyone. In other words, it is probably a normal part of the bacterial environment, or flora, of the stomach, much like the so-called friendly bacteria in the intestines.

Our industrial, postmodern society is not conducive to H. pylori. Studies show that in populations that have better hygiene and sanitation as well as smaller families, there is a lower incidence of colonization with H. pylori. (Scientists don't know exactly how the bacterium spreads from person to person.) With the widespread use of antibiotics and the concerted efforts of physicians to remove H. pylori from large numbers of people, the bacterium is disappearing in developed countries, particularly in the US.

●**Is the disappearance of H. pylori a positive development?** Yes and no. Everybody who has the organism has a condition called *chronic superficial gastritis*—a mild inflammation of the stomach that has no symptoms. However, having that condition increases the risk of developing

an ulcer by approximately three- to fourfold and stomach cancer by tenfold.

This is especially true for people who carry a strain of the bacterium called *CagA+,* one of a number of types of H. pylori. Where H. pylori is disappearing, ulcers and stomach cancer are disappearing as well. And that's good. More and more cases of ulcers are being caused by the chronic intake of nonsteroidal anti-inflammatory drugs (NSAIDs), such as aspirin and *ibuprofen* (Advil).

But as these diseases have gone away, other diseases have now become more common, particularly gastrointestinal reflux disease (GERD), commonly referred to as heartburn. In certain people, GERD leads to a condition called Barrett's esophagus (abnormal changes in the cells lining the esophagus), which in turn can lead to esophageal cancer.

In the US, the rate at which esophageal cancer is increasing is one of the fastest for all malignancies. The same is true in other developed countries, such as England, Norway and Australia.

●**Why would a decrease in H. pylori cause an increase in GERD and esophageal cancer?** With aging, there is a normal diminution in the production of stomach acid. Eradicating the CagA+ strain of H. pylori creates a biochemical process that allows the stomach to generate full levels of acid, even at age 50 and older. And it is the regurgitation of stomach acid into the esophagus that causes GERD. Additionally, studies show that there is an inverse relationship between the level of the CagA+ strain of H. pylori and esophageal cancer—those without CagA+ have a four- to fivefold higher risk of developing esophageal cancer.

●**In light of these findings, who should be treated for H. pylori?** If somebody has an ulcer, there is no question—get rid of H. pylori. The benefits far outweigh the risks. And if someone has a rare form of stomach cancer called gastric lymphoma, eradicating H. pylori is a standard part of treatment.

Otherwise, there is no reason to remove the bacteria—even though removing it, in cases of indigestion, is standard practice for many physicians. H. pylori is not a pathogen. Studies show that removing it does not improve the symptoms of indigestion.

New studies show that the stomachs of people who have H. pylori produce more leptin, a hormone that inhibits appetite. As H. pylori is being eradicated, obesity is increasing. Is there a link? Many scientists think this is a possibility.

• **If a person should be treated for H. pylori, what is the best method?** The best therapy is the simultaneous use of three or four medications, usually two antibiotics, such as *amoxicillin* (Amoxil), *metronidazole* (Flagyl), *tetracycline* (Achromycin V) or *clarithromycin* (Biaxin), an acid inhibitor (such as a proton-pump inhibitor or H2-blocker) and/or bismuth salts. The use of this combination regimen for seven to 10 days has eradication rates of higher than 90%.

Asthma Breakthrough

The medication *omalizumab* (Xolair) reduces asthma attacks by more than 50% and also allows patients to reduce use of inhaled corticosteroids, which can cause side effects. The drug, which is injected once or twice a month, is for patients with moderate to severe allergic asthma that can't be adequately controlled by other drugs.

Caution: Patients given omalizumab in clinical trials had slightly higher cancer rates than placebo patients, but the difference was not statistically significant. Patients with a personal or family history of cancer should discuss risks with their doctors.

Thomas Casale, MD, chief of allergy and immunology and director of clinical research at Creighton University, Omaha.

New Treatment for Incontinence

Urinary urge incontinence, a condition that results in urine loss before being able to get to the toilet, can be greatly eased by Milk of Magnesia.

A recent finding: Women who took one teaspoon of magnesium hydroxide—the active ingredient in Milk of Magnesia, Mylanta and Maalox—twice a day had significantly fewer episodes than those taking a placebo.

Theory: Magnesium hydroxide minimizes contractions of the bladder muscle that is responsible for an overactive bladder.

Farnaz Alams Ganj, MD, assistant professor, obstetrics and gynecology, Akbarabadi Hospital, Iran University of Medical Sciences, Tehran.

Can Earwax Removal Help Hearing Loss?

Earwax removal via a syringe can improve hearing—but not always. In a new study of more than 100 patients who visited a doctor for earwax removal, two-thirds did *not* experience better hearing after the procedure. However, in patients who did benefit, hearing improved significantly, by up to 35 decibels. Patients who do not benefit from earwax removal may be hearing impaired. They should see an audiologist for testing.

David Memel, MD, senior teaching associate, division of primary health care, University of Bristol, England.

Medical Emergency? Calling 911 May Not Be Wise

Charles B. Inlander, a consumer advocate and health-care consultant located in Fogelsville, Pennsylvania. He was the founding president of the nonprofit People's Medical Society, the consumer advocacy organization credited with key improvements in the quality of US health care in the 1980s and 1990s, and is the author of 20 books, including *Take This Book to the Hospital with You: A Consumer Guide to Surviving Your Hospital Stay* (St. Martin's).

When faced with a medical emergency, our initial instinct is to dial 911. But calling 911 may not be your only—or even your best—choice. The 911 emergency response program began in the US about 35 years ago. Most people assume that if they call 911 in response to a medical emergency, an ambulance and medical personnel will arrive in a matter of minutes. That's not necessarily true. Operators at 911 call centers are trained to assess the situation by asking the caller about the person in need, his/her symptoms, whether he is conscious, the nature of the injury and any other pertinent information that is necessary to provide the appropriate response. In some cases, such as a bad sprain or a nonlife-threatening broken bone, the 911 operator may suggest that the caller take the person to a hospital emergency room. In other instances, such as a possible heart attack, a stroke, a severe injury from a fall or a sudden severe fever in a child (above 104°F), the operator will almost always dispatch an ambulance.

Most emergency medical services units consist of an ambulance with two or more emergency medical technicians (EMTs) and, in some cases, a paramedic. EMTs receive 110 to 400 hours of training from programs typically conducted at community colleges. Paramedics have 1,000 to 1,300 hours of training, usually culminating in a two-year college degree. Paramedics are permitted to start intravenous lines, give shots and insert airway devices to assist breathing. EMTs are usually restricted to using oxygen masks and performing other noninvasive procedures, such as applying bandages or compresses.

As you can see, it's preferable to have a paramedic on the team, so check with local emergency medical services to see if the emergency response units in your area are staffed by both EMTs and paramedics. An emergency response unit is required to take the patient to the nearest or most appropriate emergency facility. The patient and family have no say in this. Each unit is in constant contact with the local hospital emergency room, notifying nurses and physicians of the patient's status.

In some cases, medical care might start sooner if you take the patient to an emergency room on your own, particularly if the patient is able to move and/or you live more than 30 minutes from an ambulance service.

Important: Arriving at a hospital in an ambulance does not necessarily mean that you'll get quicker care. Most emergency rooms make an immediate assessment of each patient and quickly move the most severe into care units, no matter how they arrived.

In many areas of the country, "urgicare" and "emergicare" centers—freestanding facilities that usually are not affiliated with any hospital—are available for minor medical emergencies, such as ankle sprains, minor rashes and sore throats. These facilities, which are typically staffed by doctors and nurse practitioners, are often less crowded than hospital emergency rooms. The centers accept most types of insurance and are usually open 12 to 24 hours a day.

Latest Research: Half of Angioplasties May Not Be Needed

Richard A. Stein, MD, professor of medicine at New York University Medical Center in New York City, and director of its Urban Community Cardiology Program. He is author of Outliving Heart Disease *(Newmarket) and a recipient of the National Institutes of Health's Preventive Cardiology Academic Award.*

Most Americans who die each year from heart disease have *atherosclerosis*, fatty deposits (plaques) in the arteries that restrict blood flow to the heart. Many cardiologists routinely recommend angioplasty (inflating a small balloon inside an artery), usually with stenting (inserting a wire mesh tube), to remove or flatten the plaques.

Newest research: *The New England Journal of Medicine* recently published a study that found that at the end of five years, angioplasty with stenting was no better than medication (such as cholesterol-lowering statins and beta-blockers to control heart rate), plus lifestyle modifications, for non-emergency heart patients. Based on these findings, some experts estimate that at least half of the 1.2 million angioplasties performed in the US each year may be unnecessary.

Surprising: The clots that cause most heart attacks usually form in areas with only minor plaques—*not* in the severely clogged areas that look so threatening on imaging tests. That's why preventing clots (by treating plaques) is actually preferable to restoring "normal" circulation to diseased arteries with an invasive procedure.

A BETTER APPROACH

Angioplasty with stenting as well as bypass surgery (grafting healthy veins from other parts of the body) can curb symptoms and prolong life when used appropriately (see "Surgical Options" on page 60).

However, researchers have found that the incidence of heart attacks in some non-emergency patients could be reduced by as much as 70% by combining nonsurgical "medical management," such as that used to lower cholesterol and blood pressure, with changes in diet and other lifestyle factors. The steps required to achieve this level of risk reduction are easy to follow—the key is simply to do *all* of them.

People who smoke should most certainly give up cigarettes. It's also important to address stress and depression—taking care of how you feel is critical to taking care of your heart. Most people know by now to eat salmon or other cold-water fish. The Harvard Physicians' Health Study found that people who eat fish once or twice weekly have a significant reduction in the number of cardiovascular events, including heart attacks.

Anyone who is at risk for heart disease (due to family history, high blood pressure or diabetes, for example) or has a history of heart disease also should be aware that...

• **Statins do more than lower cholesterol.** This family of cholesterol-lowering drugs—*lovastatin* (Mevacor) and *simvastatin* (Zocor)—has revolutionized both the prevention and treatment of heart disease. These drugs can reduce heart attack risk by up to one-third...and they're just as effective for primary prevention (preventing a first heart attack) as for secondary prevention (preventing a heart attack in patients who already have had one).

New finding: Statins may reduce the size of arterial plaques. When LDL "bad" cholesterol is reduced to extremely low levels (below 70 mg/dL), plaques stop growing or even shrink. But this isn't the only benefit. Statins also prevent plaques from getting larger...convert plaques from *vulnerable* (likely to rupture and cause clots) to *stable* (less likely to rupture and cause clots)...and reduce damaging inflammation in the blood vessels.

Suggested: An LDL reading below 100 mg/dL in patients with heart disease...or 130 mg/dL or lower in patients without heart disease. Every patient with elevated LDL should ask his/her doctor if he should take a statin. (Red yeast rice, a dietary supplement that has the same active ingredient as statins, can be taken as an alternative.)

• **Not paying attention to HDL "good" cholesterol is dangerous.** Doctors tend to focus on reducing their patients' LDL levels because there are many treatment options—and each point reduction can reduce the heart attack risk by 1%. However, HDL cholesterol may be even more important. For every point *increase* in HDL, heart attack risk drops by 2% to 3%. HDL should be 40 mg/dL or higher in men...or 50 mg/dL or higher in women.

Suggested: Taken in high doses (more than 1.5 g daily), the B vitamin niacin can increase HDL levels by 50% or more. Unfortunately, niacin at these doses frequently causes side effects, mainly itching and/or facial flushing. A slow-release form, such as Niaspan, taken at bedtime, makes side effects less troublesome. Taking a baby aspirin one hour before taking niacin also reduces side effects.

Also helpful: Regular exercise can raise HDL by about 10%. People who stop smoking also will experience a slight increase in HDL.

• **The definition of high blood pressure has changed.** High blood pressure is one of the major risk factors for heart disease. Your blood pressure should be checked by your doctor at least once a year. If it is elevated—now defined as above 120/80 mmHg, rather than above 140/90 mmHg—work with your doctor to lower it through diet, exercise and/or medication.

• **Low-dose aspirin is all that is needed.** Aspirin reduces the risk for a first heart attack by about 20%, and the risk for a second by about 25%. In patients who also have high blood pressure, it can reduce the risk for a stroke by about 35%.

Suggested: A low-dose (81-mg) aspirin daily. Higher doses are no more effective in most patients and are more likely to cause stomach upset and/or bleeding. Aspirin therapy is not recommended for women age 65 or younger who don't have heart-disease symptoms, such as chest pain (angina) during exertion. In this group, the risk for bleeding outweighs the heart-protective benefits. Talk to your doctor before beginning daily aspirin therapy.

●**Fruits and vegetables are more powerful than most people realize.** Eating nine daily servings (one-half cup each) can reduce the risk for a heart attack by as much as 30%. Fruits and vegetables contain antioxidants, which curb inflammation, and fiber, which lowers cholesterol.

Best: A Mediterranean-style diet, which consists mainly of plant foods...moderate amounts of fish and poultry...and olive oil instead of butter or other saturated fats. People who follow this diet can reduce heart disease risk by 50% or more. For more information on the Mediterranean diet, go to *www.oldwayspt.org*, the Web site of the Oldways Preservation Trust, a nonprofit food issues advocacy group.

●**Drinking wine really does help.** There's been so much talk about the heart-protective benefits of wine (red or white) that some people think it's hype. But it is true that small amounts of wine (five to 10 ounces daily for men...and five ounces daily for women) are good for the heart. Beer and spirits, in small amounts, also can be beneficial. People who drink moderately can reduce their risk for a first or second heart attack by 7% to 10%.

●**Burning up calories is more important than the type of exercise you do.** Exercise increases blood flow through the coronary arteries. The rushing blood stimulates cells lining the blood vessels (endothelial cells) and makes them more resistant to plaque buildups.

The Harvard Alumni Study looked at exercise in terms of calories burned, rather than the type or duration of exercise. Men who burned 3,000 calories a week by performing moderate-intensity exercise had the lowest incidence of heart disease. (Women should aim to burn 2,500 calories weekly.) This can be achieved by walking briskly for about 45 to 60 minutes most days of the week.

More from Dr. Richard Stein...

Surgical Options

There *are* instances when angioplasty with stenting or bypass surgery is usually necessary. These include when a patient has severe blockages in all three coronary arteries...when the heart muscle is damaged (often due to a previous heart attack)...when there are blockages in two coronary arteries...or when there's a blockage of more than 50% in the left main coronary artery. In addition, these procedures can be lifesaving if a patient is in the early stages of a heart attack or has pre-heart attack symptoms, such as worsening chest pain and/or elevated levels of certain blood enzymes.
